D1994867

Copyright © 2016 Sarah Colton

All rights reserved.

ISBN-13: 978-0692650448

Library of Congress Control Number: 2016903636

No part of this book may be reproduced in any form or by any electronic or mechanical means including information storage and retrieval systems, without permission in writing from Water Tower Books or from Sarah Colton, except by a reviewer who may quote brief passages in a review.

The actions, thoughts, and fragrance choices of real, literary, or historical characters in this book, although loosely based on fact or legend, are imaginary and fanciful, and are not meant to be taken literally.

Editor: Adelaide Farah

Cover Design: Catherine Villeminot and Pamela Paddock

Illustration: Jocelyn Haybittel Gibson

Back cover design: Catherine Seris

Aesthetic Advisor: Helder Suffenplan

To order additional copies, please contact:

www.amazon.com

contact@watertowerbooks.com

www.badgirlsperfume.com

Water Tower Books

Asheville, North Carolina 28802

USA

◈ BAD GIRLS PERFUME ◈

Tips & Tales

Sarah Colton

WATER TOWER BOOKS

2016

To the people of the fragrance community and
the wild imaginings of their spirit.

"Art is a lie that tells the truth"
Jean-Claude Ellena

◈ CONTENTS ◈

◈ CHAPTER ONE ◈

Bad Girls NEED Perfume

If you're reading these words you're already in trouble. Bad Girls are always in some kind of trouble!

Bad Girls know who they are and prick up their ears when they hear someone calling them by name.

You saw 'Bad Girls' on the cover of this book and thought, "Hey, that's me!"

But perfume? What does perfume have to do with Bad Girls?

Everything!

Perfume is made for Bad Girls because perfume is secret code for power, and Bad Girls NEED power.

You can have all the great Bad Girls intentions, plans, and agendas you want, but without power you can't make them happen, so they might as well not exist.

Power is about getting one's way. And, since Bad Girls often get their way through covert action – seduction, subterfuge, and ruse, well, that's where the specific power of perfume comes in.

When we think of perfume, we don't necessarily think of power. Instead we tend to think of seduction and desire, romance, beauty, or magic, because that's what perfume makes us see or feel. But power is what perfume is.

Perfume *powers* seduction. Perfume *powers* desire. Perfume *powers* a lot of life's experiences because it transforms feelings and perceptions. It transforms our own feelings and perceptions about ourselves, and it transforms other people's perceptions and feelings about us.

This is the essential power of perfume.

And perfumery – the entire perfume industry all the way back to the dawn of history, has been and still is, about this amazing transformative power.

◈ ◈ ◈

Let me give you an example that may surprise you.

Perfume is the *origin* of Original Sin. Believe me, I have this on the best authority. We all know the official story, and how everybody blamed Eve for making Adam eat the apple. Well, this didn't bother Eve one bit because she was a wily chick and knew everybody blames everything on women anyway. So when she, in turn, blamed the serpent, she knew full well that wasn't going to take the heat off her. Didn't matter. She did it to keep from revealing the real reason Adam ate that apple. Way too powerful a secret to share with those guys who wrote the *Bible*. But, I'm going to tell you something. I KNOW Eve's secret. It was Olfaction. The sense of smell. Fragrance. Perfume.

Olfaction, the most ancient of the five senses, is triggered in the olfactory bulb of the brain (often referred to as the reptilian brain–read *animal* here), and is at the genesis of memory and dreams. It's older and more powerful than those parts of the brain that inform us about proper conduct, law, and order.

So, here's the real story.

Adam was an ordinary man, God-fearing, obedient, and frankly dull. Eve, on the other hand, well she was a Bad Girl. For one thing, she had a huge imagination, and therefore a slightly different agenda than the one God had in mind. She knew she would have to call on one hell of a power if she was going to get Adam to do what she wanted instead of what God wanted. And this power was olfaction. Fragrance. How she knew this, nobody knows. But I'm telling you this: Eve used olfaction to bypass Adam's unimaginative brain and trick him into eating the apple. How did she do it? Simple. She just held the apple under Adam's nose and said, "Adam, Honey. You gotta just *smell* this apple!"

The rest is history. The use of olfaction, fragrances, and perfumes to transform perceptions is the oldest Bad Girl trick in the book. And it's still as powerful today as it ever was.

Not surprisingly, the savviest Bad Girls throughout history have known about this power and used it to achieve their infamous ends. Eve, of course, but also Cleopatra, Catherine de Medici, Scarlet O'Hara, and pop star Madonna are obvious examples. But there are many more that you might not suspect, such as Florence Nightingale, Hermione Granger, and The Little Mermaid.

And yes, even me, Bad Girl.

In fact, the real reason I've written this book in the first place is because the power of perfume literally changed my life. Not once, but several times. Each time it was an amazing instantaneous *transformational* experience. And each time I knew it the moment it happened.

Let me tell you a personal story about transformation....

When I was fourteen, a friend gave me a bottle of Revlon's *Jean Naté* for my birthday. The minute I unscrewed the top and smelled the fragrance I recognized myself and was transformed. I WAS *Jean Naté*.

I already was this bubbly fresh teen-age girl. But it was *Jean Naté* that set her free. Anybody who knew me at the time surely also remembers *Jean Naté*. Friends say they could always tell when I was coming, and I'm sure I overdid it, but even that wild exaggeration was an accurate reflection of my personality of the time – exuberant, fresh, and playful.

And although I didn't realize it then, *Jean Naté* was a powerful force in my life – for years. Every time I opened the bottle and smelled the fragrance it made me happy. All I had to do was breathe it in and I felt like laughing. I was obsessed with it. Bathed in it. I would have drunk it if I could have.

Jean Naté was a reflection of the over the top exuberance I felt in my teen years. Today when I look back, I smile at the thought of myself then. And I'm thankful for the fragrance that danced into my life one summer day in my early adolescence, because without my knowing it *Jean Naté* recognized me and encouraged me to be myself. And this special combination of recognition and encouragement was an enormous power that accompanied me through a wonderful chapter of my life that extended from my teens to my early twenties.

There were other fragrances I wore from time to time during those years. *CHANEL N°5*, Guerlain's *Shalimar*, and Dana's *Tabu*, are three that occasionally spoke to evolving facets of my personality. *CHANEL N°5* was the epitome of a chic and distant sophistication. *Shalimar* was voluptuousness and romance. *Tabu* was overpowering sensuality, and I would fantasize about the woman in the ad who could so distract a man that he would abruptly cease playing his violin to seize her in a passionate embrace. On occasion I would wear one of these fragrances, but they were only fleeting sentences or paragraphs in that chapter of my life. I was not yet ready for their kind of power: the edge of *CHANEL*, the mystery of *Shalimar*. And *Tabu*, passionate fantasies! It was enough to simply open the bottle and smell the cap, before quickly closing it again, throwing it in the back of my drawer, and slamming it shut. Then dousing myself in a generous splash of *Jean Naté*, I felt the perfect power for the tone and intensity of who I was at the time. *Jean Naté* was, without doubt, the name of that chapter of my life.

Sometime soon after my senior year of college I began to yearn for a different life. I wanted something else. I wanted to be somebody else. I didn't know who she was, but I could partially imagine her. She still had the zest and the energy of *Jean Naté*, but she was more worldly and sophisticated. Her energy was more focused, and her unpredictability more refined than the craziness of my teen years.

While this other person I dreamt of becoming only lived in my imagination, I occasionally caught glimpses of her, and each time she fleshed out a bit. Until one day I realized something amazing about her, or rather about her surroundings. She was in France. And I knew if I really wanted to *be* this person I would have to go out and find her where she was. By this time, she was calling me so compellingly, that that's what I did. I quit my job, left my boyfriend, and followed her to France.

And then my dream life became a tantalizing chase. I would catch glimpses of her, only to lose track of her a moment later. Reflected in ripples of the Seine; disappearing around the corner of a cobbled street in the Marais; stepping into a taxi and vanishing into the traffic at La Place de La Concorde. I even felt her sitting right next to me in a café one evening. She was *that* close.

But then I nearly lost her completely, when out of the blue my old boyfriend showed up in town. From the moment he arrived, although I knew and remembered all the reasons he wasn't right for me, I also felt the enormous and controlling power of the past. Paris and my dreams were magic and beautiful, but they were also strange and unknown.

And then one fateful afternoon, I took the opportunity to do what I love most: losing myself in this strange and beautiful city.

And it was on this particular day that I happened to walk into a Guerlain perfume boutique, and something drew me like a magnet to *Jicky*, a perfume I'd never even heard of, ironically created as a men's fragrance in 1889, and only later marketed for women. The instant I smelled it something in me cried out, "Ahhhh! That's me!"

There was no thinking. No reflection. In fact, I was so obsessed and desperate to have it immediately that I bought it on the spot, despite the major dent it put in my funds. And in this instant, my life was *transformed*. By a perfume. When I had walked into the shop I was still *Jean Naté* with all her potential, expectations, and longings. When I walked out of the shop I was *Jicky*. I had found and become the woman I had dreamt of being. The woman who had called me so compellingly from across an ocean. The woman who had made me leave everything and leap empty handedly into a world of adventure and the unknown.

My life was never the same again.

Something about the way *Jicky*'s energy coursed straight to my heart made me feel alive. It was ok to be me. Fine to be me. OMG, how thrilling it was to be me!

Immediately upon leaving the Guerlain boutique I bought myself a tighter pair of jeans, some red nail polish, and a pair of wedge-heeled espadrilles.

All the same time, *Jicky* was speaking to me on a profoundly deep level. For one thing, she got straight to the point about my relationship with my boyfriend. She didn't beat around the bush or mince her words in reminding me of what I already knew: that he wasn't right for me. And the reason was simple. He didn't love me for who I was. Instead, he loved what he wanted me to be, and it seemed that if I would only fix and smooth out a few peculiarities about myself – my naïve openness and my humor, for example – everything would be fine.

It's not like this was entirely his fault. I didn't love who I was either. I hardly knew myself. And yet I knew there was an emerging, as yet inchoate me that had been blossoming since I arrived in Paris. My dreams were still tender and vulnerable, and if I didn't believe in them enough to defend them now, they might be smothered and lost forever.

Of course, I already knew this. I'd heard myself say it a million times. But when *Jicky* said it, not with words but with the unique power of her fragrance, I felt her looking straight into places of my soul even *I* couldn't see. She saw who I was. She got who I was. And in this moment of recognition and validation, she moved me. My uncertainties about whoever the hell I was, and whatever the hell this meant were now exciting rather than frightening, energizing rather than depressing.

When I got back to the apartment, my (on the way to becoming ex-) boyfriend immediately saw the transformation in me – but it was too late. *Jean Naté* had been transformed into *Jicky* and was already flying far away from where she had been only hours before. She was clear, she was kind, she needed to be free, and now she was.

And *Jicky* had big plans. For starters, she reminded me that it was mid-July, that I was a Parisian now, and needed to leave town. Together we cooked up the idea of travelling alone to Italy, finding a small hotel in Florence, and writing for the rest of the summer.

And although *Jicky* didn't immediately tell me about Mario, the Italian with whom I would spend the month of August, something about the way she looked at me from the corner of her eye opened my imagination – and my life – to entire new worlds and possibilities.

That summer I'll never forget. The summer I first felt the

transformational power of perfume. The power of *Jean Naté* had confirmed and strengthened an adolescent girl. The power of *Jicky* transformed that girl into a woman.

◈ ◈ ◈

That was many years ago, and although I've had other transformational perfume experiences, I'll never forget the first one. In addition to the enormous pleasure it brought me, this singular experience convinced me beyond the shadow of a doubt that perfume is the most powerful ally and accomplice a Bad Girl can have.

And yet, I find it astonishing that a lot of people, including many of my Bad Girl friends who are absolute aces at managing other Bad Girl tricks, don't have a clue about the true power of perfume or how to use it for advancing their own agendas. What a waste of talent! For want of a better explanation, I sometimes wonder if this might be due to the tons and tons of academic, sometimes pedantic, explanations about perfume we hear day-in–and–day-out, making it seem so serious, complicated, and downright intimidating.

This is ridiculous. Perfume is *not* rocket science. At least, not for us Bad Girls. Indeed, the most important fact worth remembering about perfume is that *we're* the ones who invented the whole damn thing in the first place! Perfume is *our* story. Just as much a part of us as our DNA. Using perfume to carry out our Bad Girl objectives is as natural to us as any other Bad Girl things we do.

There are just a few little things to remember, tips to share, and well, tales to tell….

As a self-defined Bad Girl and journalist with more than 15 years of hacking my way through the Parisian heart of the perfume jungle, and, most importantly, as a woman whose life was transformed by the power of perfume, I've come to realize that the only thing we Bad Girls really need is a simple little inspirational book all of our own. We need to be reminded that Bad Girls have been using perfume's vast powers to accomplish their objectives forever, and that perfume is central to our illustrious Bad Girls birthright. This is simply who we are and how we operate.

And that's exactly what I've done. In true Bad Girls style I've jumped in, guns blazing, all of which has gotten me into a heap of trouble that includes writing *Bad Girls Perfume*.

Before going further, I want to make a few things clear. I deliberately do NOT define Bad Girls in *Bad Girls Perfume* beyond saying that Bad Girls define and recognize themselves. I do, however, contend that, given the primary reasons women use perfumes and fragrances (seduction, subterfuge, deception, covering up, lying, creating multiple identities, sending coded messages, etc.), at least 95% of women fragrance users are Bad Girls.

In writing *Bad Girls Perfume* I've taken inspiration from my own Bad Girl friends, including some of the most accomplished in history, literature, cinema, and the arts, who, while defying definition, are classy, discerning, and mischievous, and, perhaps most importantly, are the absolute agents of their lives and desires.

My purpose is to inspire you and all my Bad Girl friends to new levels of ace Bad Girls perfume proficiency, and to guide you to the highest caliber fragrances for the accomplishment of your most cherished Bad Girl missions.

You game? Great. Here's the deal.

First, I'm going to introduce you to some of my favorite Bad Girl friends, a personally selected team of Bad Girls Perfume mentors. They're going to tell you some unbelievably wild stories, reveal the names of their favorite Bad Girl perfumes, and the important role they played in achieving major Bad Girls objectives.

Among other things, they'll teach you basic strategies for combining multiple Bad Girl personalities ("personages") with well-chosen perfumes, while offering coaching in common, everyday, Bad Girl activities such as seduction, hunting, and banditry. They'll also suggest specific techniques for Bad Girls with special needs such as, cougars, gold diggers, mermaids, and witches. Mid-way through the course, they'll take you on a short trip to Bad Girls fantasyland, and as a grand finale (only for the bravest of the brave), they'll explore existential perfume dilemmas Bad Girls face in worst-case scenarios such as The End of the World.

And that's it, Bad Girl. After that, you're outta here.

There's nothing more to it. I'm totally confident that by hanging out with some of your most accomplished Bad Girls Perfume sisters, listening to their advice, and sharing a bunch of laughs, you'll feel totally at home, and ace the course. You might even have a *transformation*! Most importantly, you'll be ready to use the power of perfume to turn your own Bad Girls Perfume stories into the stuff of legend.

Fair warning: As you've figured out by now, *Bad Girls Perfume* is nothing less than a massive call to action. I'm not promising I'll get you out of all the trouble I get you into. But I don't think that's what you want anyway.

Are you with me? Good. Let 'er rip!

Note:

While reading this chapter, you surely noticed that I switch from third person, to first person, to second person. I'll continue to do this all the way through the book because that's the way I talk. So, don't worry about it. Sometimes Bad Girls are "you." Sometimes they're "they." Sometimes they're "me." Always and forever though, they're us!

◈

◈ CHAPTER TWO ◈

The Two Faces of Eve

For strategic purposes Bad Girls sometimes need to work covertly, and at other times it's best to work in the open. This has been the situation in Bad Girl territory since the beginning of time.

For this reason most Bad Girls have developed two opposing faces or "personas," and show one or the other to the world, depending upon the needs of the moment. There is the "Innocent Flower" persona for undercover work, and the "In Your Face" persona for work that's clearly out there. I know few Bad Girls who never, ever, switch from one of these modes to the other, although it's true that some tend to favor one over the other.

An ace Bad Girl knows that through the judicious use of a well-chosen perfume she can actually *become* whatever persona she selects for a given Bad Girl job. More than *playing* a part, she *is* this persona, thanks to the transformational power of perfume. She feels it and so does her entourage. This gives her colossal powers and separates her from all the rest.

* The "Innocent Flower" Persona

With rare exceptions, even the most brazen Bad Girls have moments when they need to come across as "Innocent Flowers," usually at times when it's necessary to impress or manipulate people who have some kind of power over them, and the best strategy is to appear sweet, vulnerable, and docile: in-laws, potential employers, career review committees, mortgage brokers, divorce lawyers, competitors, police officers, people we don't know or trust yet, all men at some point....

Throughout history, savvy Bad Girls have unerringly called upon the powers of soft pastel floral fragrances (think roses, violets, irises, peonies, freesias, and mimosas) as the perfect accomplices for this persona.

One of my favorite all-time Bad Girls, Scarlet O'Hara, is an excellent Bad Girl Perfume mentor for us all. A detailed analysis of just one of her many Bad Girl perfume exploits can be exceedingly instructive.

As you will remember from the film and book, *Gone With the Wind,* Scarlet visits Rhett Butler's jail cell immediately following the end of the Civil War in hopes of borrowing money to save her plantation, Tara. Against all odds, she has managed through grit, ruse, and manual labor, to survive the war and keep her family from starving. But now, dead broke ("cash poor" and "land rich"), she is faced with a property tax bill she can't pay. Rhett Butler, the only person she can think of with cash, is in jail at the time, and in order to carry off a successful jail visit Scarlet needs to create a demure and irreproachable lady-of-leisure persona. We see in the movie that she cleverly commissions an elegant, very proper (and alluring) dress, cut from the velvet curtains of a Tara drawing room. She even tells the prison guards she's Rhett's *sister.* What we cannot see because Margaret Mitchell chose to omit this important information from her novel, are the details about the fragrance Scarlet is wearing.

But given Scarlet's temperament and shrewdly intelligent character, it's inconceivable that she would have omitted the crucial power of fragrance from the construction of this persona. For such a pivotal "Innocent Flower" Bad Girl exploit she would have certainly chosen one of the soft floral fragrances so popular at the time, both in Europe and among upper class Americans.

Although many of these fragrances could have been procured locally, and Scarlet might have received some from other suitors, she would have cleverly chosen from among fragrances she had received as gifts from Rhett Butler. As you will remember, Rhett had made his fortune as a blockade runner (slipping through the Yankee blockade of Charleston Harbor in order to procure desperately needed manufactured goods from England and France). He was also a renowned womanizer, and would have brought back fragrances for his numerous lady friends, including Scarlet.

For the prison visit, Scarlet might well have chosen to wear a multi-floral fragrance such as Creed's *Fantasia de Fleurs* or Guerlain's *Eau de Cologne Impériale,* or she might have decided on a single floral fragrance such as Yardley's *Violet,* Floris' *White Rose,* Molinard's *Rose,* or perhaps Lubin's *Rose Liberty.* Any one of these would have sent Rhett a bouquet of important fragrance messages (softly feminine, vulnerable, faithful, and seductive).

Even in the absolute worst-case scenario in which all of Scarlet's perfumes might have been lost or stolen during the war years, she would have worn *some* fragrance, perhaps a locally produced rose or peach blossom "toilet water." In this case, her fragrance message would have been less sophisticated than that transmitted by the Europeans, but its charming simplicity would have appealed to Rhett's oldest olfactory memories grounded in his own Southern roots.

Scarlet, of course, aced the entire performance except for one tiny detail. Her hands, rough and worn from heavy farm work betrayed the lady-of-leisure aspect of her persona. Rhett was so angered by her duplicity that he threw her out of his prison cell, and Scarlet was forced to leave empty handed. BUT several days later Rhett relented and sent her a check for the money she needed. What made him change his mind? We'll never know, but it just might have been her fragrance *sillage* (the fragrance "trail" that lingers in the air or in memory after the wearer has gone).

Contemporary Bad Girls on similar missions have a plethora of fragrances to choose from, including those from large well-known brands (the kind one typically finds in department stores), as well as a growing number of less well known niche brands, sometimes referred to as "artisanal" or "creator" brands (mainly sold in specialty perfume shops).

A modern Scarlet O'Hara Bad Girl in search of "Innocent Flower" fragrances might wisely choose Yves Saint Laurent's *Paris,* with its soft and romantic message surrounded by a rosy bouquet. Or perhaps she might choose Yves Rocher's *Rose Fraîche* from the collection entitled Un Matin au Jardin (Morning in the Garden). What, indeed, could be more innocent and fresh than a rose freshly plucked from the garden? If, on the other hand, she prefers to pick her roses in the niche fragrances garden, she might try *Rose Rebelle Respawn* by A Lab on Fire, whose name speaks for itself, or she might even be so bold as to wear *I Love My Man* by Dear Rose, and let him decide whether he believes her, or not. She undoubtedly also realizes that if she wears Xerjoff's elegant and profound

Damarose with its sensual musky trail, she runs the risk of thoroughly breaking his heart.

Other soft florals presenting excellent choices include The Different Company's classy and totally modern take on the most demure of flowers *I Miss Violet,* or Kenzo's clear and innocent *Flower by Kenzo* with its gentle and powdery notes of violet, hawthorne, and rose.

In any event, having learned from past mistakes, our contemporary Scarlet would also surely plan to wear a pair of L'Artisan Parfumeur kid gloves scented with *Mûre et Musc Extrême* (blackberries and musk), and invent a plausible pretext for keeping them on during the entire prison visit – damn the heat!

For the record, several other of my favorite Bad Girl friends offer excellent "Innocent Flower" perfume mentoring examples:

Frances Stevens, in Alfred Hitchcock's 1955 suspense thriller *To Catch a Thief,* exquisitely filmed in Technicolor on the French Riviera, would have lightly but thoughtfully dabbed on Lubin's innocent green floral fragrance, *Gin Fizz,* to baffle and beguile the "Cat Burglar." (She caught him.) It helped, of course, that she did this while driving from Cannes to Monaco in her powder blue Sunbeam Alpine Roadster convertible. How do I know about her perfume? The character, Frances, was in many ways the screen embodiment of the beautiful and aloof American who played the role, Grace Kelly. *Gin Fizz* was rumored to be Kelly's favorite fragrance at the time, and as we all know, that girl knew how to use the powers of fragrance to catch a lot more than a thief.

Pour La Petite Histoire, a year later Prince Rainier commissioned the house of Creed to create *Fleurissimo* in honor of

Grace's wedding day. This "bridal bouquet" fragrance mixes pastel "undercover" florals (roses, violets, and irises) with "In Your Face" florals (mainly tuberose flowers), as well as a subtle yet very present *animalic* ambergris base note (derived from Sperm whales). Uh, oh! If there was any confusion as to what this bride was going to be up to, it was surely *his,* not *hers.*

Back on American soil, a well-advised contemporary Bad Girls Perfume friend (name omitted to protect the innocent) is adamant that I tell you this: "I know only too well that when wearing Estée Lauder's romantic and light floral fragrance *Beautiful,* I exude the essence of the perfect American *Good* Girl: fresh, squeaky clean, well-rested, and ready for the day. I can't begin to tell you the number of undercover Bad Girl successes I've achieved with this fragrance." Oooooh, that's really bad.

Another American Bad Girl friend of mine swears by Ralph Lauren's *Romance* when it comes to turning the tables on some of these guys by playing the hopelessly romantic "Innocent Flower." She thinks it must be something about the soft and rosy, yet lively and citrusy notes that give men a false sense of being in control. And yet, the truth of the matter is that they lose all sense of direction and control which just floats gently away on a peaceful cloud of violet and water-lily notes. Talk about unadulterated undercover Bad Girls Perfume power. This is it.

Other Bad Girls Perfume friends tell me they prefer to find their soft florals lurking among the shadows of the niche fragrances. In particular, several swear by the powers of Aedes de Venustas's *Oeillet Bengale.* When asked to elaborate, one such friend only laughed and said, "This undercover Bad Girl rose fragrance is so duplicitous that it hides behind the name of a carnation. "Oeillet" means "carnation" in French. And, to add yet another level of trickery, the word "oeillet" carries some wicked double meanings in French slang, ranging from intimate body parts to bra components.... I'll let you have the fun of looking this up."

Reader, take note: Bad Girls who know how to use "Innocent Flower" fragrances can get away with murder. As the unsurpassed undercover liars of perfume, pastel floral fragrances should be basic equipment in any Bad Girl's fragrance arsenal.

* The "In Your Face" Persona
There are other circumstances when Bad Girls feel, or need to act, "In Your Face." The not so subtle message being, "I'm hot and this is *my* territory. All control ends here." In my book, there are three Bad Girls Perfume "In Your Face" champions: white florals, aldehydic florals, and orientals.

* "In Your Face" White Florals
A fundamentally important thing to remember about flowers is that sweet and pretty as they appear, they're essentially the sexual organs of plants, often look remarkably similar to their human equivalents, and if you take a deep whiff (especially of those innocent looking white ones), you may be taken aback by a not-so-innocent smelling, manifestly *animalic* odor. Oooh yes! Pastel florals might be the champions for undercover work, but *white* florals crush it for "In Your Face" Bad Girl jobs.

The undisputed Queen of the white florals is the tuberose flower – primal, voluptuous, and shamelessly predatory. Gardenias, magnolias, jasmine lilies, lilies of the valley (awww, those dear little darlings – watch out!), orange blossoms, neroli (blossoms of bitter orange trees), ylang-ylang, and narcissi are also blatantly hot white florals.

To help you grasp what a hot "In Your Face" white floral fragrance can do, think of that uber pop star, professional Bad Girl, Madonna – in real life, or in just about any of the characters she's ever played. Full-bodied and voluptuous, Madonna could be the poster child for Robert Piguet's fragrance, *Fracas,* an over-the-top tuberose "In Your Face" white floral. In French, *Fracas* means "a noisy disturbance or quarrel."

Madonna has reportedly worn *Fracas* (created in 1948 by the perfumer Germaine Cellier, another notorious Bad Girl) on many occasions on and off stage, and even claimed it as one of her favorite fragrances. That is, until 2012 when she launched her own signature white floral tuberose fragrance, *Truth or Dare* by Coty, which some say smells scandalously similar to *Fracas.* Oh, la-la. What a Bad Girl, Madonna! But that's another story.... The important thing about *Fracas* is that it shouts *strong sexual presence.* Not every woman can manage *Fracas.* Think of it as the fragrance equivalent of snap your fingers, quick nod to the band director, entrance music. You've got to have, or be ready to assume, the attitude, "Yeah, this is the real thing, sucker. Get yourself an eyeful while you can!" as you enter a room, all the while relishing the audible gasps from the parting crowd.

Madonna, of course, didn't invent the wheel for exploiting tuberose fragrances, which, of course, has been spinning pretty much out of control ever since Bad Girls began walking the planet. Another excellent example of tuberose power comes from just over a century ago in the person of Jane Avril, the beautiful and talented French Can-Can dancer of 19th century Belle Epoque Paris. Made legendary by the art deco posters of one of her lovers, Toulouse Lautrec, Jane shared a special

Tuberose Secret with her fellow dancers, all of whom, like herself, were seasoned Bad Girls by character, as well as by profession. Living as they did, by their wits on stage and off, these girls knew a thing or two about the specific powers and usages of this most formidable floral. An important secret shared among them for keeping their wealthy lovers was the application of a tiny drop of tuberose oil in those places on their bodies – mounds and crevasses – where they wanted to be "explored."

Modern perfumery offers plentiful tuberose fragrances for similar exploratory purposes. Jeroboam's sultry and white-hot tuberose fragrance, *Hauto* created for contemporary Bad Girls with similar "In Your Face" fragrance needs, calls on the spirit of Jane Avril, her fellow Can-Can dancers, and their fragrances. Another powerful secret weapon tuberose fragrance is Nasomatto's *Narcotic V* which is nothing short of the addictive intensity of female sexual power.

Frédéric Malle's tuberose fragrance *Carnal Flower,* clearly takes enormous pleasure in flaunting the juicy curves of her Bad Girls body in a sheer gown of exotic flowers and white musk, and is known for her crowd stunning "In Your Face" maneuvering.

Using an entirely different strategy, Histoires de Parfums' *Tubereuse 2 Virginale* is an unmerciful tease. Classy and smooth skinned with the softest of cherry lips, she creates unbearable desire by revealing only a hint of her tuberose charms, while keeping the rest tantalizingly out of reach.

It's true that white florals, and in particular Tuberose fragrances, can be daunting at first, and Bad Girls looking for a way to discreetly wade into tuberose territorial waters without throwing everything completely off balance might consider a fragrance I like to think of as a "tuberose light" (although many might say that's a contradiction in terms). Maria Christofilis's *Fleur 09* is just that. Approachable though distinctively tuberose, this fragrance is, in fact, a highly qualified double agent. Soft and clean-smelling on first whiff, it draws your victim in for another go, all the while allowing you to get closer to your target undetected. Be careful, though. Nothing provokes more charged emotions and fire than a double agent revealed, so you might want to practice this at home. OMG! Did I just hear myself telling a Bad Girl to *practice* something before flinging herself headlong into the fray? In any event, fair warning: not for the faint hearted.

Tuberose, of course, is not the only "In Your Face" white floral with a knockout punch. Bad Girls have played other white florals since the dawn of time, with earth-shaking consequences. Indeed, it could be argued that the Sexual Revolution which defined the entire second half of the 20th century and is still going strong in the 21st, was triggered by a single white floral perfume in the hands of a very, *very* Bad Girl. Oh, yes. In spite of everything you might have heard about the important role patchouli fragrances played in ushering in the era of free love, wait just a minute and listen to what I'm telling you. When Brigitte Bardot burst onto cinema screens as the character Juliette, in Roger Vadim's 1956 film *Et Dieu Crée la Femme (And God Created Woman),* she literally embodied what was to become an entire generation of sexually empowered flower children. Juliette/Bardot's youthful, pure, and blatant sexuality was so powerful that even she couldn't manage it, and essentially drove every man in her life to distraction. Her fragrance? Ah, but of course, and *mais oui!* It could have been none other than Christian Dior's *Diorissimo,* a single floral lily of the valley fragrance created by one of the greatest perfumers in history, Edmond Roudnitska, in the same year as the film.

More than a half-century later, an accomplished Bad Girl can have just as much fun and raise as much havoc, by delivering Juliette's trademark Bad Girl double whammy "In Your Face" *hot* and *out of control* message to any and all ill-fated victims who might penetrate her territory. For starters, she knows how to create a totally fictitious sense of peace and feminine wholesomeness by spritzing her personal space – car, office, living room, boudoir, etc. – with Frédéric Malle's *1er Mai,* a fresh and vegetal lily of the valley home fragrance, dispensed via a "perfume gun," yes, that's what it's called. Then, to finish off the job, she simply douses herself generously in another lily of the valley fragrance such as, État Libre d'Orange's *Don't Get Me Wrong Baby, I Don't Swallow.* Pandemic insanity guaranteed.

For Bad Girls with an orange blossom bent, Cuban-American designer Narciso Rodriguez's modern, sexy, indeed blatantly lustful, *Narciso Rodriguez for Her* literally exudes open and deliberate "In Your Face" carnal desire with its powerful orange blossom, musk, and amber notes. Not surprising that it was created by one of the hottest perfumer teams ever to come together on a 21st century brief: Christine Nagel and Francis Kurkdjian.

Meanwhile, some of my Bad Girl friends prefer the refreshing and slightly bitter bite of neroli, and swear by the virtues of Lisa Hoffman Beauty's *Tunisian Neroli,* both for the lush and intoxicating quality of the fragrance and for the variety of ways they can wear it, including as jewelry. But that's another story. Suffice to say that this rich and sensual fragrance, and the design concept that accompanies it are made for Bad Girls, perhaps because they were designed by someone who should know, the wife of one of Hollywood's most iconic Bad Boys. I'm here to tell you, this Girl knows a thing or two about perfume power!

Hearts leap at the glorious trumpeting notes of Le Labo's elegant and soaring *Lys 41,* as the ravishing and mischievously spicy Lily makes her entrance accompanied by "In Your Face" Jasmine and Tuberose. Indeed, it's only thanks to the softening influence of Vanilla and Musk that adoring fans, instead of dropping dead on the spot, simply swoon and and live to tell the tale. And what a tale – memories and dreams of a moment's heady spectacle, forever etched in the annals of Bad Girls Perfume history.

If gardenias are what turn you on, you should definitely consider Jovoy's shamelessly uncorseted and "In Your Face" fragrance *Gardez-Moi,* for Bad Girls Perfume missions in the wild and desperate spirit of the Roaring Twenties. For missions of a more subtle tone, especially those requiring the wearer to work in darkness, Tom Ford's heady and complex *Velvet Gardenia* is decadent and *animalic.* (Unfortunately, this fragrance has been discontinued so you may have to sleuth around for it on e-bay.)

For the Bad Girl magnolia fans among us, Julian Bedel's *Agua Magnoliana* offers the "In Your Face" headiness of a flirtatious magnolia blossom shamelessly dancing in a fragrant breeze of sandalwood. And by all means, don't shrink from the Down-Under niche brand Grandiflora's opulent *Magnolia Grandiflora Michel.* If Grandiflora knows something about magnolias, it stands to reason that perfumer Michel Roudnitska, son of the perfumer who gave us Dior's havoc-wreaking

Diorissimo (as witnessed earlier in this chapter) would know something about white florals. He does. Heady, complex, and ripe, *Magnolia Grandiflora Michel* is a voluptuously meaty floral fragrance, languidly perfuming and caressing the breeze.

Fair warning, narcissistic Bad Girls may get themselves into more trouble than they bargained for with Caron's shifting and conflicted *Narcisse Noire,* as you'll find out soon enough in Lara's story recounted in Chapter 8: Make War, Not Love. Meanwhile, Thierry Blondeau's *Narcisse Émoi* is totally effective, and doesn't pull any punches with its out-there and edgy citrusy leather interpretation of the narcissus flower.

Jasmine lovers know and cherish the numerous qualities of this small and delicate flower, and rely on the many faces she can assume. In Serge Lutens' *À La Nuit,* Jasmine gathers the immense diversity of her family and brings in Indian, Egyptian, and Moroccan cousins to offer a multi-layered sensuous fantasy of languid summer evenings beneath a canopy of stars.

Meanwhile, in État Libre d'Orange's *Jasmin et Cigarette,* jasmine presents a completely different face. There's nothing soft about this red-lipped Bad Girl, strong, confident, and brassy, who prefers hanging out with the tobacco and leather crowd in stilettos and mini-skirts.

As for lush and tropical Ylang-Ylang, she's a totally unpredictable Bad Girl who seldom acts alone, and can show erratic behavior depending upon the company she keeps. In Annick Goutal's *Passion* for example, Ylang-Ylang and her "In Your Face" cronies, Tuberose and Jasmine, are blatant Bad Girl Teasers. While allowing themselves to be fondled by Bad Boy Vanilla's warm and velvety touch, they keep the rest of their offering fulminating and tantalizing just out of reach. By contrast, in By Kilian's *Voulez-Vous Coucher Avec Moi* (Do you want to sleep with me?), Ylang-Ylang doesn't mince her words one bit, and is clearly *out there* aided and abetted by her "In Your Face" white floral pal, Tuberose, and warmed up by her intoxicating accomplice Vanilla. Meanwhile, her quietly seductive friend, Bulgarian Rose, simply sweetens the offer by displaying the softness of her curves.

As for Ylang-Ylang's behavior in Maison Francis Kurkdjian's wild and intense, *Absolue Pour Le Soir,* she's so totally pumped up by her entourage, including that Bad Boy, Benzoin, that she WILL not be contained for love or money.

Jean Patou's classic 1930 masterpiece *JOY,* offers every Bad Girl the perfect juxtaposition of equal doses "Innocent Flower" rose, and "In Your Face" jasmine, for a continuous flip-flop of patent contradictions. In one instant she's clearly the sweet and docile rose, and in the next she's the totally hot and out of control jasmine. This fragrance experience can really make people lose their minds. Only temporarily, of course, but just long enough for Bad Girls to accomplish their objectives.

Bad Girls whose strategies require a bit of stealth will totally appreciate the disarmingly lovely fragrance bouquet of Prudence Paris's *Nuits Blanches* (Sleepless Night) which carefully integrates (hides) "In Your Face" white florals among "Innocent Flower" pastel florals. Needless to say, this fragrance is highly recommended for tricky agenda items requiring camouflage, disguise, and other surprise tactics.

Another highly recommended and unusual stealth tactic perfume arrives from the exotic Indian sub-continent in the guise of Neela Vermeire's *Pichola.* In this mesmerizing and startlingly beautiful fragrance, "In Your Face" tuberose and orange blossoms approach as if in a mirage, reclining in voluptuous splendor on the backs of elephants, and drifting on a cloud of exotic Indian spices and warm woods.

In yet another Bad Girls mixed message bouquet, April Aromatics' *Lindenblossom* (Unter den Linden) weaves the soft romance of a summer evening's stroll under the linden trees in Berlin, with just a hint of "In Your Face" magnolia as a reminder that the night has not yet revealed all her charms.

A contemporary libertarian Bad Girl might enjoy the mixed message she creates hiding her game (at least for a while) in the rosy heart of Lubin's 2016 fragrance *Upper Ten for Her,* while occasionally letting a charming little hiccup escape from its base notes of raspberry liqueur.

Meanwhile, Bad Girls who prefer to mix their white florals in more traditional arrangements can accomplish all their objectives clad in nothing more than Givenchy's sweet and classic *Organza,* which like a fluid and translucent dress is draped in sensual folds of gardenia, tuberose and jasmine, and softly belted in warm vanilla.

Considering the extraordinary powers of all these White Floral "In Your Face" fragrances whether working solo or in gangs, be sure to use them with ~~caution~~ abandon.

* "In Your Face" Aldehydic Florals

Unlike other florals, aldehydic florals don't grow on trees. Nor do they grow in gardens. As their name indicates, aldehydic florals incorporate one or several synthetic molecules known as aldehydes in their formulas, and are therefore at least partially the fruit of the human imagination. Although known for the variety and intensity of their smells, aldehydes are especially appreciated in perfume compositions because of their capacity to enhance and boost the fragrance and diffusion of other raw materials in a formula, for a "shimmering" and "effervescent" delivery.

First isolated at the turn of the 20th century, aldehydic molecules were hot *avant-garde* items in perfumery during the early1920s, and clearly caught the eye of Mademoiselle Coco Chanel, just as she was coming up with the idea for her now legendary 1921 fragrance, *CHANEL N°5.*

Among other things, she wanted her perfume (primarily composed of equal parts rose and jasmine) to be expensive and unique. As anybody knows, Bad Girls don't like half measures, and true to form, Coco Chanel, didn't ask her perfumer Ernest Beaux, to just experiment around a little bit with a small percentage of aldehydes. She told him to pour it on.

The result was the groundbreaking fragrance whose dazzling initial impression is often compared to champagne because of its shimmering top notes.

It didn't take long for Bad Girls from around the world to pick up on the scent of *CHANEL N°5,* recognize it as a first class Bad Girls Perfume, and start putting it to use for their wicked purposes. Of the numerous Bad Girls Perfume stories and legends this fragrance has engendered, my favorite comes straight out of a well-known chapter of literary history. Though, of course, not officially documented, I do have it on the best authority that during the infamous literary summer of 1922, a certain Mrs. Daisy Buchanan was most surely wearing the recently launched *CHANEL N°5.* She was impressed by the stir the fragrance had already created in the glitzy Jazz Era world she inhabited, and in true Bad Girls style, Daisy wanted to test its effects on her personal entourage. In particular, she wanted to try it on a man people called Gatsby. The Great Gatsby. Anyone who's read F. Scott Fitzgerald's 1925 book or seen the film, knows that the effects were devastating for the totally unsuspecting Gatsby, who was most definitely stirred,

indeed seduced, by the whole production. Poor
the very first instant, he never had a chance. Indee
totally befuddled that even when Daisy insisted up ng
his Rolls on the way home from a boozy party, he acquiesced. Later when he took blame for the fatal car accident, the fate of this man was sealed. Ah, the nefarious powers of perfume!

And there are many others. In the next chapters of *Bad Girls Perfume,* we'll follow the infamous exploits of other notable "In Your Face" aldehydic floral fragrances. Indeed, you may be shocked to learn, for example, that Lanvin's *Arpège,* Dolce & Gabanna's *D&G,* Jean-Louis Scherrer's *Scherrer 2,* and Andy Tauer's *Noontide Petals* are incomparable seductresses; that Rochas' *Madame Rochas,* Paco Rabanne's *Calandre,* and Yves Saint Laurent's *Rive Gauche* are scheming thieves; and that Le Galion's *Sortilège,* Lancôme's *Magie Noire,* and Cacharel's *Loulou* are sagacious witches. Prepare yourselves.

* "In Your Face" Orientals

Orientals are the other reigning champions of "In Your Face" Bad Girls perfumes. Hot and sultry, these fragrances are dominant and overpowering, typically smelling of resins, vanilla, incense, spices, amber, and oud. With no middle ground, their message is either Strong Positive, as in, "Come here, *now!*" or Strong Negative as in, "Steer Clear! Too hot to handle!" Or, more devastating still, both at the same time, as in "I know I shouldn't tangle with this one, but OMG, I can't resist!" Oh yes. "In Your Face" Bad Girls know that one of the most important purposes of oriental fragrances is to excite, confuse, and ultimately exhaust their lovers.

A "Who's Who" of world-class oriental fragrances would certainly start off with great 20th and 21st Century fragrance classics such as, Coty's *Emeraude,* Guerlain's *Shalimar,* Estée Lauder's *Youth Dew,* Yves Saint Laurent's *Opium, Giorgio Beverly Hills,* Dior's *Poison,* Calvin Klein's *Obsession,* Beyoncé's *Heat,* Serge Lutens's *Féminité du Bois,* and Tom Ford's *Black Orchid.* Along with white floral and aldehydic floral fragrances, these "In Your Face" oriental fragrances heat up and cause trouble for anybody who comes near them, as you'll soon see.

Bad Girls have been using "In Your Face" oriental fragrances since way back. Don't forget, some of the best Bad Girl mentors in history come to us straight out of the *Bible.* The Old Testament *Book of Judges* tells us about Delilah who cajoles her lover, Samson, to reveal the source of his colossal strength, and then betrays him to his enemies. In the New Testament both Matthew and Mark tell us about Salome, who so enchants Herod with her erotic dancing that she's able to make him give her the head of John the Baptist on a plate. And yet, nowhere in these accounts is the power of fragrance evoked. Surprise, surprise. These Bad Girls weren't born yesterday. Taking their cues from Eve before them, they knew better than to give their secrets away to a bunch of men, and preferred to leave coded hints for savvy Bad Girls, *laid* between the lines. The reference to "The Dance of Seven Veils" in the Salome story is one of these hints, and opens our eyes to something Middle Eastern Bad Girls have practiced for centuries: "layering." Similar to the "layers" in "The Dance of Seven Veils," both Delilah and Salome would certainly have practiced layering with their fragrances. Starting with ritualistic bathing and cleansing with fragrant oils (musk, oud, rose, orange blossom, jasmine…), they would then infuse their hair, clothing, and personal spaces with fragrant burning incense, all of which would fall into the modern day category of "orientals." Make no mistake, Salome's veils and Delilah's pillows, in addition to being seductive in color, texture, and drape, were profoundly perfumed.

Contemporary Delilahs and Salomes have an unprecedented array of fragrant "oriental" products which, when layered, can create highly personalized perfume experiences as powerful as "The Dance of Seven Veils." Layers can be on a single theme, such as Francis Kurkdjian's *Lumière Noire,* which weaves oud, cedar wood, patchouli, and saffron into a room spray, a candle, and a scented body cream. Or, for rich harmonies and subtle contrasts, Bad Girls can mix and match layers by choosing products such as Aqua di Parma's *Oud* shampoo, Tom Ford's *Oud Wood Bar* soap, Serge Lutens' *Ambre Sultan* EdP, or the countless charms of Annick Goutal's *1001 Ouds.* Or to get straight to the point, they can simply apply Byredo's *Seven Veils* to each and every layer.

A story told by one of my favorite contemporary Bad Girl perfume friends, let's call her Nikki, illustrates the hypnotic and totally obsessive effects of orientals, and their power to transport us over time and space. Now, Nikki's a California Bad Girl, and all I have to do is mention the name *Giorgio Beverly Hills,* and she's gone. GONE! In less than the twinkling of a mischievous eye and what I would swear is a rush of wind in her hair, she's suddenly far off. I'm not sure where, but this Bad Girl is driving. Sometimes she's flying along the Pacific Coast highway. Sometimes she's cruising downtown LA. It's 1981, Nikki's an ambitious 22, and has just landed her first job in a hot LA PR firm. "The first thing I did," she tells me, "was what *anybody* would do, darling. I bought myself a little red Mercedes convertible to scoot around town in. For business, of course, but that always rhymed with pleasure–and with *Giorgio.*

"All part of the memory. The first moment I smelled *Giorgio's* voluptuous flowery oriental notes I started obsessing and thinking, wow, now that's a rich girl's perfume. You've got to picture it. I know it sounds insane, but my very first whiff of *Giorgio* came to me as this intoxicating fragrance billowing out at me from my mailbox. I didn't know what was happening. Turns out, some (other) brilliant PR person had thought to include a sample of *Giorgio* with my subscription of *Vogue.* And not just mine. In cities all across America. Talk about out there. Imagine. Women everywhere, opening their magazines, and POW! Of course, this kind of marketing became common practice right after that, but *Giorgio* was the first fragrance to do it, and this was key to its amazing and instant success. People literally went crazy over *Giorgio.* Oh, man, that's exactly what happened to me. *Giorgio* immediately became *my* fragrance. Everything about *Giorgio* was me, and not just its outrageously flashy fragrance. Here I was, this nouveau rich *Babe,* and *Giorgio* literally shouted sex and money. And to top that off, it was called *Giorgio Beverly Hills,* inspired by the famous Giorgio boutique, and packaged with the distinctive yellow and white striped frontage of the retailer on LA's Rodeo Drive.

"Not to brag, but *Giorgio* and I were hot. I was going somewhere, and anybody who wasn't already there, or getting me there – I just left them behind in a cloud of dust. So much fun accelerating away from a stop light at the intersection of Hollywood and Vine. Of course, since the top was down the whole time and the wind kept blowing my *Giorgio* off, I just had to keep applying it so I could keep obsessing. When I think back, I'm sure it was overpowering. W-a-a-a-y over the top. But then, so was I."

Editor's Note: As of this writing, nothing has changed.

Fair warning: Before applying an oriental fragrance, be sure to calibrate the dose to your intended message. Following the launch of Giorgio in 1981, restaurants across America posted signs saying, "No Dogs! No Cigars! No Giorgio!"

Before leaving this chapter, and I probably shouldn't tell you this because it really is dangerous stuff, but my Bad Girl friend, Juliet, insisted. Speaking across centuries with the legendary authority of one of the greatest romantic heroines of all time, Juliet was adamant that fragrances adept enough to encompass the duality of Bad Girls' "Innocent Flower" "In Your Face" nature, are more precious than life itself. How else to endure the heavy passion of a love like hers for Romeo and the feather-light innocence of those same feelings. Among such rare fragrances available today, Juliet keeps a special place in her heart for the *Far from the Balcony* collection by the brand Giulietta Capuleti, which takes us beyond the stereotype of a fifteen-year-old romantic heroine to the very soul of a tenacious and determined young woman, courageous enough to choose the singular path of her own destiny.

◈

◈ CHAPTER THREE ◈

The Seductress

Seduction is hands down the most effective way for a physically weaker person (i.e., a woman) to get what she wants (power) from a physically stronger person (i.e., a man).

Through the art of seduction, the "weaker" person makes the "stronger" person (willingly and pleasurably) give his power away. Although this might seem to contradict what I said earlier – that nobody willingly *gives* away power – the truth is, power isn't given away for nothing. It's given in *exchange* for something else.

When you get down to it, men are pretty basic creatures with predicable responses to given stimuli, so that "something else" most commonly associated with seduction is sexual favors, the promise of sexual favors, or more often than these guys would ever think (don't tell), the mere *suggestion* of sexual favors.

Not surprisingly, seduction is the central driving force in many Bad Girl schemes, and perfume, that most powerful and invisible suggestion of sexuality, plays a central role.

We saw what Eve was able to accomplish with Adam, using "nothing" but the fragrance of an apple. And though it's true that over the course of centuries, women and perfumes have evolved to bring remarkable complexity and subtleties to seduction, the male of the human species has evolved very little, thus, that "something else" of the basic seduction exchange has remained virtually unchanged.

Similarly to Bad Girls changing personas, seduction follows a continuum from subtle, coy, and (seemingly) passive, to upfront, shameless, and (unmistakably) active.

At the passive end, *existential* seduction, whether innate or carefully contrived, is sufficient unto itself, has the mesmerizing energy of hot embers, and communicates in presence, attitude, and subtle movements of posture, eyes, or lips.

At the active end, *operational* seduction is raw and unadulterated, has the high energy of combustion, and communicates through dramatic movement, song, dance, and sweat.

* Existential (Passive) Seduction

Bad Girl Marlene Dietrich (1901–1992), the mysterious and mesmerizing German-American actress is a perfect embodiment of existential seduction. In spite of a look that contemporary Bad Girls may find dated, she managed to transform her inborn talent for seductive pouts and moues into the stuff of legend, on and off screen. Doubtless, the cunning Marlene and the characters she played cultivated this image with equally seductive fragrances.

As Lola Lola, the cabaret singer-dancer in her first film *The Blue Angel (1930),* I'm convinced that Dietrich would have been wearing Coty's *Chypre* when she seduced Immanuel Rath, the esteemed old bachelor and professor at the town's university. Poor, hapless Professor Rath. Neither he nor his reputation ever recovered. Nobody disputed the fact that Lola Lola had her charms. But surely it took something more than this to drive a paragon of academic restraint and discipline so irredeemably over the edge.

Bad Girls, of course, know the answer. It was her fragrance, *Chypre,* arguably THE definitive seductress fragrance, created in 1917 by one of the most gifted perfumers of all time, François Coty. Both groundbreaking and earth shaking in its precise formulation built around a sharp contrast of citrus and floral notes with a woody, oak mossy accord, *Chypre* is warm, dry, animalic, and perilously sexy.

Named after the island of Cyprus (Chypre in French), renowned for its fragrances throughout antiquity, Coty's now legendary fragrance, *Chypre,* was to engender an entire family of fragrances, duly entitled "chypres," which includes such greats as Guerlain's *Mitsouko,* Dior's *Diorama,* Weil's *Zibeline,* Carven's *Ma Griffe,* Hermès *Calèche,* Ungaro's *Diva,* Schiaparelli's *Shocking,* Robert Piguet's *Bandit,* and *CHANEL N°19.* You'll be seeing plenty of these Bad Girl chypre perfumes in action soon enough in subsequent chapters of *Bad Girls Perfume.* Meanwhile, don't be thrown off by their languid and sultry personas. Behind the façade, these Bad Girls are extremely hard workers.

Though often misunderstood, chypre fragrances speak to the very soul of Bad Girls – strong, complex, sensual, and unstintingly committed to their cause. Depending upon their makeup, chypres can work both "Undercover" and "In Your Face," and can include a variety of floral, fruity, woody, and leather notes. Perhaps most importantly, once a chypre fragrance has become your ally she will never let you down.

In the course of my career I've noticed that many of my Bad Girl friends are reticent about chypre fragrances, perhaps because they sometimes come across as being too heavy or complicated. If you're in this group, I strongly recommend that you make friends with at least one chypre fragrance. Although it may take a bit longer than with fragrances of other families, you won't regret it. *Au contraire,* it may change your life. And who knows? It might even cause a transformation.

Indeed, as a contemporary Bad Girl Seductress you can do just as much damage as Lola Lola did to Professor Rath with the help of some well chosen modern chypre fragrances, most of which are considerably lighter than the traditional classics, while still maintaining their complexity and depth.

The ultimate Parisian in its studied nonchalance, CHANEL's warm chypre fragrance, *31 rue Cambon,* carries the unspoken minimalist codes of the chic city dweller so central to Coco Chanel and her brand. As easily wearable as a perfectly structured CHANEL jacket, its green and citrusy shoulders are pared down at the waist with a touch of black pepper, and while its heart notes of iris, rose, and ylang-ylang whisper of impeccable bloodlines, it ultimately and discreetly gives in to base notes of patchouli and labdanum.

Serge Lutens' dark and *animalistic* chypre, *Rose de Nuit,* recalls the shadowy and abstract image of a rose as remembered from a walk in a garden on a sultry summer's evening. Sisley's *Soir de Lune* is the irresistible attraction of a mysterious yet magnetic stranger under a moonlit sky, and Aqua di Parma's tender and romantic *Iris Nobile* clings to the skin like an ardent lover.

Bad Girl Seductresses, venturing into chypre territory for the first time will be pleasantly surprised by James Heeley's *Hippie Rose* a totally *fun* chypre, thanks to its playful and funky throw-back hippy rose-patchouli notes. Wearable and seductive, *Hippie Rose* promises flowers in your hair and the easy hedonistic pleasures of Free Love.

The Bad Girl Seductress sure of her game and ready for a modern take on a classic chypre, should be forewarned that by mixing her own inimitable talents with the sharply contrasting masculine and feminine *animality* of MDCI's *Chypre Palatin,* all players will inevitably cede to the irresistible call of carnal desire. By all means, take the plunge!

Having learned the virtues of oriental fragrances for "In Your Face" Bad Girl activities, you may be surprised to learn that oriental fragrances are also excellent for seemingly more "passive" existential Seduction. The reason may lie in the appeal of contrasts between the two extremes. An excellent example is the successful use Marlene would have surely made of Corday's masterful oriental fragrance *Toujours Moi* (Forever Me), in the 1932 film *Shanghai Express.* As the renowned prostitute, Shanghai Lily, Marlene surely and purposefully would have counted on its obsessive vanilla and erotic amber notes in the final scene. Having worn *Toujours Moi* years previously to successfully convey her absolute faithfulness to her lover (in the face of more than convincing evidence to the contrary), she could be sure that he would never doubt her again.

Modern Bad Girls on old-flame seduction missions, listen up. NOTHING is more powerful than perfume to deliver an intact, if ever so softy "air brushed" memory. Here's a challenge: Invite Salvatore Ferragamo's warm and voluptuous oriental fragrance, *Golden Acacia,* to accompany you on a daring Bad Girls Perfume mission in which you revisit the scenes of a long ago summer romance in Tuscany – Florence, the hills of San Gimignano, the beach at Piombino. Might your Italian lover still there? Might he still be hoping you'll come back? Waiting for you to come back? You'll never know unless you go. And if he is, he too may capture the shimmering perfumed glints of golden memories. Outcomes may be intense.

Greta Garbo, another European (Swedish) seductress and beauty, four years Dietrich's junior, set Hollywood on fire with an equally rare talent of bringing an entire screen (and its viewers) alive by the tiniest movement of head, eyebrows, or lips. There can be no doubt that she, too, relied on seductive fragrances to complement her enormous talents.

Starting with her very first MGM hit, the 1926 film *Torrent.* In this story, social and family obligations in the lives of star-crossed lovers, Leonora Moreno, aka La Brunna, and Don Rafael Brull, stand off with the equally powerful forces of what can take place in the seductive and fragrant shadows of an orange grove. There can be no doubt that Leonora's perfume throughout the film would have been Guerlain's radiant yet velvety soft 1912 oriental masterpiece, *L'Heure Bleue,* with its whispers of neroli, the blossom of the bitter orange tree.

If Garbo were to remake *Torrent* today, she might choose Prada's sophisticated *Infusion de Fleur d'Oranger* whose stunning orange blossoms are enhanced by tuberose and jasmine. Alternatively she could choose Vero Profumo's *Rubj* (Pronounced "Ruby") in which orange blossom notes are paired with a down-and-dirty cumin note. In either case, I'd be willing to bet money that Don Rafael would stand up against his mother's wishes this time, and our dear Bad Girl Sister Leonora could finally enjoy the pleasures of her career *and* her lover.

In later films such as the 1931 *Mata Hari,* in which Garbo plays the infamous World War I spy and double agent, I imagine she would have worn Lanvin's 1927 aldehydic floral fragrance, *Arpège,* whose mixture of both "Undercover" and

"In Your Face" floral heart notes is more than capable of betraying even the most skeptical of lovers. Contemporary Bad Girls on similar double agent missions would do well with Dolce & Gabanna's first fragrance, another quite intensive aldehydic floral, *D&G,* of sharp and alluring contrasts – sweet and bitter, feminine and masculine. Meanwhile, Jean-Louis Scherrer's elegant and conplex aldehytic floral *Scherrer 2* is capable of capturing suspecting and non-suspecting victims in dense amber layers of seduction with just enough brightness from fruit notes to show how irredeemably lost they are. And not to be denied are the powers of yet another aldehydic floral fragrance, Andy Tauer's *Noontide Petals,* whose mixture of "Undercover" and "In Your Face" heart notes seems to shimmer with life and glamour. Nobody will ever want to doubt your word.

Meanwhile, my Bad Girl friends agree that Garbo would have worn Houbigant's bright and worldly totally Bad Girl floral bouquet fragrance *Quelques Fleurs L'Original* during the production of the 1932 film *Grand Hotel.* And I'm talking about the entire thing–pre and post–production. She not only seduced her leading man, John Barrymore, but the jury for the Academy Awards, as well. The film won the Oscar for that year's Best Picture. Directors, producers, and hopeful ingénues take note.

Although known for her famous quote, "I want to be alone," Garbo knew very well how to stir up her fans. On more than one occasion her very presence at film premieres caused near stampedes in waiting mobs. Even police officers in charge of maintaining order were so visibly stirred that they were of little use in containing the crowds. Contemporary Bad Girl Seductresses ready to let loose Garbo style stampedes of avid fans, should think carefully before applying *Misia,* CHANEL's floral bouquet of ultimate feminine glamour from the Les Exclusifs collection. This supposedly "Innocent Flower" fragrance (including powdery violet, iris, and rose notes) elicits "In Your Face" emotions, perhaps because it speaks directly to profound memories of feminine accessories such as face powder and lipstick. By now, I know it's useless to suggest that you be careful, so just be ready. Check your lipstick, powder your nose, and by all means wear the right shoes!

Beyond all doubt, one of the world's greatest Bad Girl Seductresses on and off camera was Marilyn Monroe. Given her considerable talents, Marilyn could wear anything or nothing and still succeed in whatever Bad Girl Agenda item she undertook. As proof, she was the first major Hollywood star to get away with posing nude while at the height of her career. Although much has been written and surmised about her personal fragrance choices, she did, on at least one occasion, brag that she bathed in *CHANEL N°5,* not surprisingly a floral aldehydic fragrance.

From husbands Joe DiMaggio and Arthur Miller, to the President of the United States (and *All the President's Men,* apparently) Marilyn seduced more than a generation of men AND women. In addition to other seductress fragrances I imagine she would have taken naughty pleasure in wearing (at least second hand) *Eight & Bob,* a rare and confidential woody and sensual men's fragrance, discovered by young Jack Kennedy during a visit to France in the summer of 1937. Upon request, Albert Fouquet, its creator, made up a special batch for Jack, eight of his buddies, and his brother, Bob. Had Marilyn not died tragically at the age of 36 in 1962, she would certainly have enjoyed re-living many a scandalous memory through the renewed life of the same fragrance, re-launched in 2012 by the brand that now bears its name, Eight & Bob.

Another scandalous seduction takes place in Patricia Highsmith's 1950's novel *The Price of Salt.* Brought exquisitely to life in the 2015 film *Carol,* starring Cate Blanchett as the beautiful and sophisticated Carol Aird, and Rooney Mara as Therese Belivet, an aspiring young photographer. At one point, Therese recalls the very instant the seduction took place – when Carol walked into the toy section of the New York department store where she was temping. Was it happenstance that Therese also noticed Carol's perfume within this same moment?

Later, over a first lunch, a second cocktail, and a closer whiff of Carol's dusky and faintly sweet fragrance, Therese fantasizes of thrusting the table aside and burying her face in Carol's scarf.

Powerful stuff, this fragrance. Chances are high it was Guerlain's temperamental if peach-skinned chypre fragrance *Mitsouko,* a masterpiece of mystery and sophistication. Granted, its wearer is Carol/Cate Blanchett, perhaps at her most alluring moment in the entire film.

As the story evolves it becomes clear that the seduction is not simply a one-way affair. Carol is clearly moved by Therese's youthful openness that seems to have been "flung out of space." I can easily imagine Therese wearing Pierre Balmain's green floral fragrance, *Vent Vert,* a whiff of delicate yet resilient young life, bursting to be free, and suggesting the first breeze of spring.

A contemporary Carol, like her 50's sister, would surely choose a chypre fragrance, as well. For evenings, I imagine her wearing Clinique's floral aldehydic chypre, *Aromatics Elixir,* a legend in American perfumery, bold and confident, yet also hidden and private. By day, I picture her in The Different Company's *Sublime Balkiss,* which like Carol and the Queen of Sheba for whom it is named, is beautiful and mesmerizing in its Bulgarian rose, Egyptian violet leaves, and lilac heart notes, yet wise and mysterious in its patchouli and leather base notes.

In touching contrast, a contemporary Therese would be drawn to *avant-garde* fragrances among the niches. Given her interest in photography she would first be drawn to the name of Ulrich Lang New York's vetiver musk fragrance, *Aperture,* before immediately snapping awake to the edgy beauty of its focus. In other moments she would find comfort and inspiration in Nomenclature's *Adr-ett* (meaning "neat" or "dapper" in German), a spare and smartly trimmed fragrance built around the synthetic musk, Helvetolide, which gives off a softly enveloping aura of otherworldly stillness and weightlessness.

* Operational (Active) Seduction

A prime example of wildly out there, Active Seduction comes surging from the wilds of Iberian Andalucía bearing the name of Carmen. One of the strongest European archetypes of hot-blooded Bad Girl Seduction, Carmen and her sister spirits have sparked collective fantasies and imaginations since the dawn of time.

Brought vividly to life in painting, music, dance, and literature, Carmen continues to find flesh-and-blood manifestation in women of Latin temperament throughout the world. Like perfume, Carmen's volatile energy is augmented – even ignited – by certain fragrant materials. Historically a feral and untamable gypsy girl, Carmen would have enhanced her natural powers of sensuality by perfuming her hair, body, and clothing with crude artisanal fragrances and homemade concoctions made from flowers and oils native to Andalucía – orange blossoms, roses, lilies, carnations, and amber.

Contemporary Carmens can choose from a wide array of explosive fragrances inspired by her energy. In addition to white floral and oriental fragrances, first-rate chypre fragrances can spring from the shadows to "Out There" seduction in less than a most passionate heart-beat.

Paloma Picasso's signature chypre fragrance, *Paloma Picasso,* resonates with the natural *terroire* of the Carmen myth. Like the mezzo-soprano voice of Carmen in Georges Bizet's 1875 *opera comique,* the harmonies of Paloma Picasso's fragrance are provocative, seductive, and dominant, asserting an earthy, not feminine but *female* sensuality.

Lurking behind the soft woody notes of Molinard's *Habanita* are all the requisite "Out There" floral and amber notes necessary to take on even the most strenuous of seduction jobs. *Prends Garde à Toi* (watch out) by the brand Ego Facto, seduces and enlivens with a troubling and explosive mixture of masculine and feminine energies in its woody and jasmine notes, and its surprising touch of stinging nettle can keep even the most ardent suitors on their toes. *Seville à L'Aube* (Seville at dawn) by L'Artisan Parfumeur is a "no holds barred" hot oriental orange blossom fragrance of passion and desire, with just enough of the darkly spiritual to transform the untamed heat of the Carmen story into the stuff of a complex modern-day legend.

Meanwhile, the universal appeal of wild and untamable gipsy energy has inspired fragrances around the world. From Sweden, Byredo's *Gypsy Water* sings of the heat and earthiness of the gypsy girl through its woody and aromatic notes, while

Suleko's *Djelem* is the unbridled joy of the impulsive gypsy spirit of Russian lore, evoking bright colors, wild dancing, songs, tears, drinking, and, ultimately, exhaustion.

From Sicily, Ortigia Sicilia sends us darkly sensual *Ambra Nera* (Black Amber), surging with the bright fulgurating plants and herbs of her island, hot like the blood of her notoriously passionate people. And from Argentina via Italy, the warm and spicy amber notes of *Tango* by Masque Milano, set the stage for yet another dance of Latin seduction: A mid-summer night, a bower in full bloom, wooden tables, liquor… and music.

Not to be outdone, America's woody and leather chypre fragrance, *Azurée,* by Estée Lauder, takes Carmen's seduction message WAAAY OUT THERE IN YOUR FACE, while Sarah Horowitz's powerful fragrance, *Lioness,* leaps from the *animalic* depths of Bad Girl Seduction.

A word of Caution for Carmen Bad Girls:

Tragically, Bizet's Carmen didn't listen to the words of her own aria, *L'Amour Est Un Oiseau Rebelle* (Love is a Rebellious Bird), in which she warns her lover of the mortal dangers of her charms, and to *Prends garde à toi!* (Watch out). Upon learning that Carmen has left him for a glamorous toreador, he kills her in a fit of jealous rage.

I know any suggestion I might make to Bad Girls that seduction fragrances be used with caution would be like waving a red flag in front of a *taureau.* For the record, allow me to repeat the words of Carmen's own haunting refrain, *Prends garde à toi!*

◈ CHAPTER FOUR ◈

~~Beg, Borrow, or~~ Steal

Excuse me! Beg? You've got to be kidding. Borrow? Don't think so. Steal. Ahhhh! Now, that's Bad Girl territory. Don't get me wrong. I wouldn't *really* steal something any more than you would. Unless, of course, for some arbitrary and unjust reason it had somehow gotten into the wrong hands:

–A fabulous jewel languishing in the possession of a malevolent despot.

–The man of my life, trapped by the mesmerizing spell of a malicious rival.

–Cars, clothing, accessories, perfumes, *attitudes* that have somehow been unrightfully demarcated as "men's territory."

Restoring a captured diamond to its rightful owner and stealing my man back from that slut, who in the most underhanded way snaked him away from me, are totally justifiable, commendable, indeed statutory, Bad Girl theft and duty. As for petty thievery, anybody knows that's just the way Bad Girls stay in shape. After all, Bad Girls are anything but bad sports! Whatever the booty, and whether calling for intricate cloak and dagger intrigue with disguises and scripts, or a (supposedly) impromptu full frontal surprise attack, such as tossing a glass of champagne in that thieving bitch's perfectly made up face, the right perfume is the indispensable accomplice.

No matter what kind of stealing we're up to, elegantly cool jobs in the dark of night, or hot steamy affairs carried out in broad daylight, we absolutely must know which perfumes we can rely on in times of greatest need. As we will see, some theft accomplice fragrances have years of notoriety and are well known in the *milieu*, while others are new on the turf and eager to establish their reputations.

* Grand Larceny

The Doyenne of doyennes for grand larceny fragrances is Robert Piguet's *Bandit*. Of all the fragrances that excite this category, *Bandit* stands out as the elegant and enigmatic *grande dame* of the wicked, and reminds us that our dark side should be lived with class and verve. Launched in 1944, *Bandit* was the creation of perfumer Germaine Cellier, a Bad Girl in her own right, as mentioned in Chapter 2: The Two Faces of Eve in connection with another of her notorious fragrances, *Fracas*. Needless to say, Germaine and her perfumes were very VERY Bad.

As my own first acquaintance with a perfume on the dark side, *Bandit* initially attracted *this* Bad Girl with nothing more than the power of her name, sultry green bottle, and vintage photos of the dagger flashing models at her initial launch. But as soon as *Bandit* began whispering her delightfully wicked leather chypre notes to me from the shadows, I knew beyond all doubt that she was my best accomplice for any job taking place under cover of darkness. Faithful, stealthy, tireless, and now over 70, this Bad Girl *Bandit* is still brandishing knife blades and stealing the show.

In the 1964 dark-ish comedy, *Topkapi,* Elizabeth Lipp (Melina Mercouri) is the personification of Grand Larceny Banditry at its best. We can literally feel *Bandit's* chypre intensity emanating from her olive skin, husky cigarette voice, and deeply mascaraed eyes as she ring-leads an ambitious though ill-fated jewelry heist from the Topkapi Palace museum in Istanbul. Throughout the film, our Bandita heroine maintains the ironic humor of the perfect Bad Girl Bandit, even when faced with the abject failure of a stint in prison (largely due to the blunderings of her male accomplices). Undaunted, our heroine is already plotting her next heist. Hard to keep a good Bad Girl Bandit down!

Another Bad Girl Grand Larceny film of the same era is Blake Edwards' 1963 comic masterpiece *The Pink Panther.* Though supposedly starring Peter Sellers as the bumbling Inspector Clouseau, David Niven as Sir Charles Litton, the infamous and debonair gentleman jewel thief, nicknamed "the Phantom," and a beguiling Pink Panther cartoon character, the film is totally dependent upon the unstinting undercover work of several Bad Girl perfume stars and their human accomplices. Posing as a minor character in the film, for example, Inspector Clouseau's oh so innocent and proper (looking) wife Simone (played by the actress Capucine), was doubtless working hand-in-glove with Rochas' fruity chypre fragrance, *Femme.* It's not like you haven't been warned, guys: *Cherchez la Femme!* Where else could Simone have found that *je ne sais quoi* of feminine energy so necessary for maintaining not one, but *two* lovers, occasionally even hiding them in closets and under beds. The exiled and seductive Princess Dahla (Claudia Cardinale) was surely working closely with another Bad Girl fragrance, the sultry, floral, and aldehydic chypre *Calèche* by Hermès, as she stole a few hearts, the show, and… perhaps even, the diamond….

Ah HA! Who really stole the pink panther, that mega-carat diamond with a central flaw resembling a panther? Hard to tell in the confusion of a masked ball and bewildering fragrance clues left by an assortment of likely and unlikely suspects. There were many who accused Clouseau himself, who disguised as a knight in *rusty* armor, would have left an inimitable *sillage* of the spicy fougère aftershave, Mennen's *Skin Bracer.* Surprisingly, nobody suspected Sir Charles, assuming, perhaps erroneously, that a man wearing Acqua di Parma's *Colonia Acqua di Parma* is beyond reproach. And it goes without saying that nobody seriously thought it was the zebra, although some complained of suspicious and quite *animalic* fragrance droppings near the scene of the crime. Most highly suspicious of all was the pair of mirror image gorillas lurking around the vault where the diamond was hidden, and I'm here to tell you they were absolutely wearing Comme des Garçons *Guerrilla 1* and *Guerrilla 2!* Perfectionists might find this troublesome, given the fact that this insane fragrance duo had not yet been created at the time of the film. Just goes to show that everything is possible with Bad Girls Perfumes.

In all seriousness, no one knows who really stole the Pink Panther. Was it *Jolie Madame* by Pierre Balmain, *That Man* by Revlon, or, who knows? Maybe, *It's You* by Elizabeth Arden. I'm not telling....

Not to worry. The Pink Panther was to strike again on numerous occasions and for many years, offering more intriguing and hilarious mysteries to solve, while continuing to delight fans, until the premature death in 1980 of the actor Peter Sellers brought an abrupt end to the merriment. Even so, sometimes in dreams and fantasies I catch glimpses of the charmingly eccentric buffoon, Inspector Clouseau, and other zany characters from the series, and imagine them brought to life again by the miracle of modern perfumery. Starting with Clouseau's wife, Simone, that Bad Girl jewel thief and femme fatale. I know she's wearing Ann Gerard's "Innocent Flower" fragrance *Rose Cut* as she continues to plot even more diamond heists with her favorite accomplice, none other than Sir Charles Litton, who in his gentlemanly perfection is wearing Houbigant's impeccably modern classic, *Cologne Intense.* Meanwhile, the Princess Dahla remains her seductive self while wearing the sultry and spirited oriental fragrance, *Epic Woman* by Amouage, while the inscrutable Clouseau is wearing Antonio Alessandria's woody and spicy *Nuit Rouge,* as he continues to wreak mayhem in his relentless search for the Pink Panther. As my fantasy continues to unfold, the fabulous costume party is still in full swing with the same bewildered zebra trotting about, this time, actually wearing a fragrance, Jovoy's *Lys Epona,* with its unusual mix of lilies and a surprisingly pleasant and tenacious "barnyard" trail. Oh yes, and the twin gorillas are still at it, although strangely enough they no longer seem to care about finding The Pink Panther. Mainly, they're just insanely happy to finally be wearing their falsely eponymous fragrances, Comme des Garçons *Guerrilla 1* and *Guerrilla 2,* which having waited more than 40 years, have at last emerged from the shadows of perfume creation to greet them.

Fifty years later, a 21st century Bad Girl Pink Panther reveals herself, though reluctantly at first, in the 2013 British film, *Love Punch.* Like many Bad Girls at some point in their career, the film's heroine, Kate Jones (Emma Thompson), is so undercover that even *she* doesn't know it. Sound familiar? Not a problem. Can happen to the best of us.

Turns out, this handicap is only transitory for Kate thanks

to a basic quirk in her Bad Girl nature, which, surprise, surprise, includes a strong sense of fairness – especially when self-interest is involved. Indeed, motivated by nothing less noble than the call to mete out Bad Girl justice, Kate embarks on an adventure that initially leads her into lots more trouble than she intended (maybe).

Fragrances to the rescue. Thanks to the skilled deployment of several high caliber perfumes (typically left out of the movie script), along with a bit of creative genius for setting things straight (another Bad Girl quirk), Kate manages to land on her feet, recover the iconic jewel (of course, there's a jewel), and not inconsequentially, get her man back. Not bad, considering that the particular man in question is played by none other than Pierce Brosnan.

Based on meticulous sleuth work, I've uncovered serious evidence that Kate's primary perfume accomplice in the film is *Velvet Rose & Oud,* a versatile, seemingly unassuming fragrance by Jo Malone, which *mine de rien,* is adept at playing both ends of the Bad Girl game (read "double agent"). Highly discreet, yet well-known and respected in the *milieu,* this floral oriental fragrance is deceptively unassuming (at first), and is capable of sneaking up from behind a totally Undercover Bad Girl façade to softly pounce like a cat burglar. Really bad!

Not surprisingly, Kate only feels *Velvet Rose & Oud's* "In Your Face" jolt after she's left her comfort zone of suburban London, and jumped into the "Out There" universe of Paris' Left Bank, where even hotel-keepers and their perfumes are drop-dead sexy. After that, it doesn't take much to trigger our bad girl to "In Your Face" action. Indeed, four little words, "the flame still burns!" are all it takes – uttered, as it turns out, by none other than one such drop-dead sexy hotel-keeper, brilliantly played by Marisa Berenson. Berenson, of course, could be wearing nothing other than *Shocking,* the scandalous signature fragrance of her maternal grandmother, the fashion designer Elsa Schiaparelli.

From this moment on, Kate and *Velvet Rose & Oud* are masters of every conceivably Bad Girl trick from kidnapping and gatecrashing to grand larceny and cliff hangings. At a crucial point Kate and *Velvet Rose & Oud* even feign a parting of the ways, just long enough for *Enigma,* a musky *animalic* oriental perfume by Roja Dove, to provide Kate with the necessary ground support to carry out a daring mission into totally wild Bad Girl Cougar territory.

The final scenes of the film show Kate re-united with her ex-x-husband, whose fragrance, Mont Blanc *Legend,* has apparently won out. Of course, any Bad Girl worth her carats can see from a new look in Kate's eye, that her current "Undercover" persona is merely the façade of a thoughtfully calculated "safe house," in which she's running a tidy little *ménage à trois* with *Velvet Rose & Oud* as her primary accomplice, and *Enigma* close at hand for whenever the need might arise....

* Take the Cash and run

Bonnie Parker, made legendary in American pop culture by Arthur Penn's 1967 film *Bonnie and Clyde,* starring Faye Dunaway and Warren Beatty, was a tough and resilient Bad Girl, willing to kill when necessary, and with a carnal weakness and romantic soft spot for Clyde Barrow, her lover and partner in crime. She was also surely a desperate fan of *Evening in Paris* perfume. In the years 1931 to 1934, as half of one of history's most famous "Public Enemy" duos, her moments between robbing banks were few, but I'm sure like any woman,

Depression years or not, Bonnie dreamt of strolling into the local Woolworths, hanging around in the cosmetics aisle, maybe even lingering over a Coca-Cola at the soda fountain. Chances are, her real shopping trips took place at a faster clip, with a sheriff hot on her heels. More of a chase than a stroll, Bonnie would have been forced to exercise a hasty five-finger discount as she grabbed up the items on her shopping list, including, of course, a quick bottle of *Evening in Paris*. At home that night she might obsessively smell this soft and classic sweet floral fragrance, and quiet her sleep with dreams of a real *evening in Paris,* and of calmer times, lulled by floral notes of violets, clover, lilac, roses, and jasmine. On occasion, she might even test its effectiveness on Clyde.

Ironically, perhaps because of its years of easy availability in dime stores across America from the 20s to the 60s, *Evening in Paris* is often misunderstood as a cheap and ordinary fragrance. *Au contraire!* Known as *Soir de Paris* in France, it was created in 1928 for the brand Bourjois by none other than Ernest Beaux, one of history's greatest perfumers, the nose behind *CHANEL N°5* and other CHANEL masterpieces.

Why would Bonnie have chosen *Evening in Paris?* She didn't have time to tell me. I sometimes wonder though, if in her southern heart she harbored dreams of an early retirement to violets, roses, and clover. Or, given her personality and the demands of the job, it might well have simply been the cobalt blue *bullet-shaped* purse flacon, briefly on the market from the 20s through the 50s, which first caught Bonnie's eye and spoke to the free and reckless spirit of a girl.

◈ ◈ ◈

* Revenge: 'Hell hath no fury…'

Ooooooh! Revenge is one of Bad Girls' favorite tricks and, in my opinion, much more fun and challenging than simple jewel thievery, and even tops grand larceny. Bad Girls are first and foremost players. Props and disguises. Schemes. Laying traps. Acting out. Creating drama. Manipulating. Spying. Heating emotions past the boiling point. Anger. What could be more motivating than a desire for revenge? And nothing could be a better partner in crime for revenge than perfume.

Bad Girls driven to the limits of insanity by unfaithful partners might dream about the kind of revenge only possible for the likes of Nancy Archer in *Attack of the Fifty Foot Woman,* a 1958 B rated cult film starring Allison Hayes. Imagine the superhuman power of Nancy, a Californian heiress and beauty, who following a close encounter with an alien space ship receives a dose of radiation which makes her grow overnight into a 50 foot giantess of colossal strength.

Now that's the kind of larger than life power Bad Girls dream of. Enraged by her husband's infidelity, she now has the size and strength to do something about it. Just to make her point and grab everybody's attention, she starts off by wreaking holy havoc around town, striding through the streets crushing all beneath her feet. She then rips the roof off the building where her cheating husband is carousing with his conniving girlfriend. How she manages after this is not a pretty picture, but the fact remains: she does "get her man back" in the end.

What earthly fragrance could have accompanied such fantastical powers? Perhaps, *Enchanting Menace* by Evyan, an obscure and now defunct American fragrance and brand of the same era as the film. Like Alice in Wonderland after eating the mushroom, our Bad Girl giantess would have had to grab it quickly as she shot past the height of her dresser in her growth spurt. We'll never know the true potency of *Enchanting Menace* as it has subsequently been discontinued ... perhaps it was TOO powerful.

Not to worry. Bad Girls in similar situations and in need of extraterrestrial perfume strength might consider exposing themselves to Thierry Mugler's *Alien.* Launched in 2005, *Alien* is more often described as a powerful feeling than as a smell. In addition to its warm, dry, and very strong jasmine and woody notes, many women claim to smell quirky (what would you expect for the creator of *Angel ?*), harsh, and rough edged notes including gasoline, burning hair, nail polish remover, and even Windex. Heck. Whatever works.

Bad Girls in the mood for less violent retribution, such as a bit of harmless hair pulling, or innocently tossing a glass of champagne in a rival's *hateful* face, can find plenty of motivation in one of my favorite Helmut Newton photos. Although this photo has an official caption (see below), I prefer to call it "Elegant Champagne Toss in the Face of That Bitch and Hated Rival," which for me says it all. The Official caption is "Two beautiful women eye each other wickedly, wearing the famous Lurex pullover with chains that the young Azzaro created for [Israeli singer and writer] Rika Zaraï. The woman in the white pillbox hat has just thrown her drink into the face of her rival in the black pillbox hat!" Nova, April 1973. Photograph by Helmut Newton. © The Helmut Newton Estate/ Maconochie Photography.

I first discovered this photo gem within the pages of a fabulous little book containing photos Newton took for iconic Bad Boy fashion designer, Loris Azzaro, and I have to tell you, it was a one of the inspirations for writing *Bad Girls Perfume.* Something about it just set me off, perhaps because it captures and illustrates an exemplar "Undercover" Bad Girl in action. I'm telling you right now though, this photo only tells part of the story, as you'll soon see.

Both women in the photo are dressed to kill – not a hair out of place, high-end, classy. And yet, seething just beneath the surface of one of these Good Girl façades is the capacity to do something so wickedly funny that it can only be successfully carried out at close range. And here, yet again, the power of perfume comes into play. Our Bad Girl would definitely need something covert in order to approach her rival undetected. The wrong perfume would give her away long before she could get this close.

Considering the time and circumstances of this photo, I'd be willing to bet one of those Lurex pullovers that Loris Azzaro created his 1975 signature fragrance *Azzaro* with this Bad Girl's stealth needs in mind. Ultra-sophisticated and guileful, like our champagne tossing Bad Girl, this woody chypre fragrance also has a wicked sense of humor. Unfortunately, it's been "discontinued" (code for hiding out underground), so if you're bent on finding a bottle your best bet would be to research some "safe houses." Hint: start with eBay. Or, who knows? Maybe your mother has some. The likelihood increases if, like our Bad Boy Loris, she has Sicilian blood. If all else fails, *Azzaro Couture,* the 2008 (family successor) of the fragrance, or even *Azzaro Pour Elle* will certainly do in a pinch.

Did I hear somebody say "pinch"? OMG! I swear the thought never crossed my mind. But now that you mention it, it's just *too* tempting. I mean, God only knows when another such opportunity might present itself.... So, thinking quickly now, if I time things right, all I have to do after first applying a discreet drop of *Azzaro,* is approach my target within an appropriate distance, toss my champagne in that odious woman's hateful face, and yank at her dyed-and-sprayed-to-within-an-inch-of-its-life hair. At this point, she'll surely lurch forward, and all I'll have to do is reach behind and....OUCH! (As far as I know, Helmut Newton never captured this moment in a photo. Please, someone prove me wrong!)

Another excellent Bad Girls stealth perfume is By Killian's *Good Girls Gone Bad* which opens all fresh and innocent with an excellent and rosy "Innocent Flower" facade, before revealing its true intentions, brilliantly orchestrated by two great masters of "In Your Face" maneuvers, tuberose and narcissus.

The Bad Girl drama queen who prefers to act out her revenge on center stage, will surely find moral support and might even take a few cues from Ungaro's Bad Girl floral aldehydic chypre fragrance *Diva.* Still another great fragrance for a center stage "In Your Face" Bad Girl is *Mad Madame* by Juliette Has A Gun. Playful and explosive, this fragrance leaves absolutely no doubts as to what her intentions are (certainly not noble), and says to hell with what anybody says about her, just as long as lots of people are saying it.

Meanwhile, when it gets to down and dirty, you can't beat Gucci's *Envy* for a Bad Girls revenge mission motivated by jealousy and anger. Green, lascivious, *animalic* and potent, Gucci's *Envy* will agitate and provoke your most primal territorial juices to the boiling point, and the *sillage* (trail) will linger long afterwards like a deeply satisfying sigh of "Mission Accomplished!". Editor's advice: You girls play *nice,* now.

◈ ◈ ◈

* Petty Thievery

As much as I love grand larceny and revenge, I end up spending a lot more of my time engaged in petty thievery. Men's stuff, mainly. Great fun and plenty of booty. I notice a lot of my Bad Girl friends doing this too, almost as compulsive behavior. It even seems it's not so much the man they want, as his possessions and power. Some of the easiest and most fun kind of petty thievery is going after show-stealing articles of clothing. Leather motorcycle jackets and tuxedos are hot items on Bad Girl off-the-cuff it lists these days. Other popular plunder items include accessories and gadgets, fragrances, cars, attitudes, and entire belief systems that have somehow been unrightfully demarcated as exclusively "men's territory." Not surprisingly, there are specialized fragrances for accompanying these not always innocuous forays into male territory.

Here's the fact of the matter: ace Bad Girls recognize petty thievery as essential for keeping warmed up and toned, and they practice it daily. Innocent enough, you might think, but beware. You can catch a lot of heat for this kind of activity. You *are* stealing fire from the Gods, you know, and mocking a basic territorial urge, to boot. Additionally, since Bad Girls practice petty thievery with a *je ne sais quoi* of sizzling femininity, interactions can become "heated." Which of course, makes it all the more fun to carry off.

The most brazen trick, of course, is to take whatever it is you've stolen, and imbue it with your own style, morphology, and, of course, fragrance *sillage,* so as to leave only tantalizing traces of its ever having belonged to anyone else. Carrying this off calls for daring, wit, and the most subtle sleight-of-hand, but isn't that what gentle[wo]man burglary is all about?

Starting with the most obvious, certain fragrances that have originally been marketed for men can do amazing things for women. I've already told you how Guerlain's *Jicky* worked a transformation in my life. More recently, *Special For Gentlemen* by Le Galion spoke to me in similar ways, and for some reason, as in the case of *Jicky,* I didn't realize it was a "Men's" fragrance until I read the label. Duh. Just goes to show that labels, and in particular, gender attributions, can sometimes be misleading. Current wisdom might suggest that an elderly gentleman in my childhood wore these fragrances, and I [mis] took his power for my own. In my Bad Girls Perfume heart of hearts I believe the reasons might be darker. Or, maybe I was just born to be a trespasser. Speaking of which, when wearing Imaginary Authors' self-proclaimed post-modern fragrance, *Memoirs of a Trespasser,* a perfume of hallucinatory inventiveness, I have the sneaking suspicion that somebody, I won't name who, has been reading my diaries. Memo to self: Change password.

Meanwhile, stolen articles of men's clothing such as jackets and trousers, shirts, coats, hats, and ties are great show stealers, and perfumes are Bad Girls' perfect accomplices for all such operations. I can assure you, for example, that on at least one occasion, the crisp dry vetiver notes of CHANEL's *Sycomore* were responsible for the heist of a freshly starched pleated evening shirt, while the bright metallic notes of Yves Saint Laurent's *Rive Gauche* pushed me to steal the silver studs and cufflinks to go with it. Once I had gone this far, fantasies about Arquiste's delicate and buttery lapel gardenia, *Boutonniere No.7* incited this Bad Girl to go for the whole damn thing, and "borrow" the evening tails, as well. The party was great!

Having come this far, the only logical next step is to steal the poor guy's entire wardrobe. Yves Saint Laurent's collection *Le Vestiaire des Parfums* even stipulates which items to filch: *Caban* (Pea-Jacket), *Caftan, Tuxedo, Saharienne* (bush jacket), and *Trench.* And when it comes to THE trench, Burberry's *My Burberry* is the perfect fragrance to inspire and carry off such a *coup*. Definitely an "Innocent Flower" fragrance aided and abetted by the added illusion of a London garden in a soft spring shower, absolutely nobody will suspect as you slip into this most coveted item before quietly disappearing into the crowd on the high street.

At the end of the day, few articles of men's clothing are more comfortable for casual sleepwear than the supple knit of a borrowed and generously sized polo shirt, and more than one Bad Girl has discovered how much she loves waking and realizing she spent the night dreaming in a pleasantly hazy residue of man odors and the spicy grassy notes of *Ralph Lauren Polo.* If in addition to this, she's somehow gotten mixed up in Ramon Monegal's *Cotton Musk* (so far, no explanatory details have been offered here) she claims the memory is further heightened by the odor of soft cotton sheets.

God forbid, but should there be any dirty linen at the conclusion of this entire sordid affair, the astute Bad Girl knows she can entrust it all to the fragrant fabric-care products of *The Laundress New York,* and walk away smelling like a rose.

When it comes to poaching in that wonderfully sexy zone of male territory where leather, suede, and tobacco products converge, it's hard to beat Caron's 1919 elegant libertine fragrance *Tabac Blond,* a landmark Bad Girls Perfume for almost a century now. More recently, Carner Barcelona's *Cuirs,* recalling the fragrance of freshly tanned leather in artisanal ateliers, as well as Naomi Goodsir's *Cuir Velours,* with its absolutely decadent blend of tobacco and the suppleness of leather, will totally provoke your desire to pilfer all leather goods, from brogues and bomber jackets to bigger stuff like club chairs, and – why not? – the sumptuous driver seats of cars, speedboats, yachts, and airplanes. For Bad Girls craving the very softest, most subtle of suedes, Keiko Mecheri's floral chypre, *Lady Pointe,* turns thieving into an art as the graceful interplay of dark mosses and incense, juxtaposed with light florals and cistruses, create similar contrasts to the soft nap of the coveted material. Meanwhile, Bad Girls whose leather fetishes fixate on objects in warm Havana brown and tobacco tones, tell me that Patricia de Nicolai's *Cuir Cuba Intense* enlivens the senses and focuses the mind.

Not to be ignored, the high drama recounted in Imaginary Authors' fragrance, *The Cobra and the Canary* is full of decadent tobacco and leather notes mixed in with those of fast cars, racetracks, and cocktails. Just a reminder that the art of clandestine Bad Girls Perfume thievery is the stuff of hot and sexy spy thrillers.

Meanwhile, a high powered Bad Girl friend of mine, bent on stealing a sumptuous leather embossed seat on a (formerly) all male executive committee, told me that *1 Million* by Paco Rabanne was just the ticket to the boardroom. This, of course, makes me think of the legendary *perfume brief* for one of Paco Rabanne's all-time great perfumes, *Calandre.* It supposedly read something like this: "…a man picks up his girlfriend in his Jaguar XK-E, they take a drive beside the sea, then stop in a forest and make love on the hood of the car." I've discussed this titillating proposition with countless Bad Girls, and although reactions have been varied and sometimes even quirky, everyone agrees on one thing: Whatever your position, apply your perfume strategically and remain firmly in the driver's seat.

Bad Girls for whom the sky is no limit for pilfering expeditions, the undeniable sex appeal of airplanes can prove to be irresistible. Fortunately there's Guerlain's 1933 fragrance, *Vol de Nuit* (Night Flight), dedicated to the exploits of intrepid pilots in the 1920s and 30s, including none other than Amelia Earhart, Bad Girl aviatrix model *par excellence,* and interloper in this nearly exclusive airborne men's club. Amelia and her plane tragically disappeared forever in 1937 while on a bold attempt to circumnavigate the globe. But the balance of dark leathers and woods with the luminous orange blossom and narcissus notes of this legendary fragrance will forever recall the soaring and indomitable spirit of this Bad Girl heroine, and inspire future generations to challenge even the powers of the God Apollo for ownership of the skies. A modern Bad Girl aviatrix of similar valor would do well to set her compass points on the green and metallic notes of adrenaline-filled *Aviation Club* by Quebec fragrance brand, Monsillage.

* Power and Self-Esteem

"Face it, girls. I'm older and I have more insurance!" This throwaway quote from the 1991 film, *Fried Green Tomatoes* brings us to another important territory traditionally reserved for men: Power. Not to be excluded from the coveted objects of Bad Girls thievery are big and small manifestations of power, such as leading one's own life, speaking one's mind, driving fast cars, swearing, buying one's own perfumes, etc.…

Face it, girls, nobody is going to give power away. If you want it, you've got to go out and get it. And believe me, this is one sure way to become, and become known as a Bad Girl.

Three strong anti-heroine Bad Girls animate the film *Fried Green Tomatoes* (inspired by the 1987 novel of the same name by Fannie Flagg), which spans the time between the Depression and the 1980s in the deep South.

Octogenarian, Ninny Threadgoode (Jessica Tandy) whiles away the hours in an Alabama retirement home with racy stories about Idgie Threadgoode of the Whistle Stop Café, and captivates the imagination of her new forty-something friend, Evelyn Couch (Kathy Bates).

Unbeknownst to all but the very savvy, fragrances guide and support these Bad Girl characters throughout the entire film.

While the young and feisty Depression era Idgie (Mary Stewart Masterson) of the story would have turned up her tomboy nose at the idea of wearing any perfume, she would have loved wearing her friend, Brady's prized bottle of Dana's *Canoe* cologne. In addition to using this clean and spicy fougère fragrance as a coolant (more about this in Chapter 9: Cool Under Fire) Idgie would have worn it as a trophy to taunt Brady, having won it from him in a poker game (fair and square), a fact that totally infuriated him and, of course, made him fall even more (hopelessly) in love with her.

On at least two occasions, however, Idgie would have put aside her rebellious principles long enough to apply some soft floral "Innocent Flower" fragrance, perhaps Avon's 1925 *Lilac Vegetal.* She would have done this before serving up an unusual, but quite tasty Bar-B-Que to an extremely suspicious detective at the Whistle Stop Café, and later when she had to appear in court before an all-male jury on a charge of murder. The Bar-B-Que received compliments, and the jury pronounced her "not guilty." Thank you, Bad Girls Perfume!

For her part, dear Mrs.1980s Threadgoode of the retirement home is one of the most spirited and young-hearted Bad Girl octogenarians I've ever known (besides my own mother), forever upbeat and positive. I'm absolutely certain her perfume would have been *Charlie!* by Revlon, a bright and bubbly floral-aldehyde fragrance launched in 1973. Mrs. Threadgoode would have loved the lively magazine and TV ads starring Shelley Hack, the first fragrance advertising campaign to show a woman wearing pants (trousers for my British friends). AND it was the first fragrance specifically created to be bought by women for themselves, instead of for men to buy for women. Despite the fact that *Charlie!* was marketed for a 30s-something career woman, Mrs. Threadgoode would have declared, "That's for me!", and arranged for somebody to drive her to Belk's to get it. Knowing Mrs. Threadgoode, I'm sure she would have liberally shared it with all the nurses and CPAs on the staff, for the amusement and inspiration of all. Indeed, thanks to Mrs. Threadgoode, the halls of her retirement home would have been redolent with the bright and uplifting notes of *Charlie!*.

It's not surprising that Evelyn, inspired by her growing friendship with Mrs. Threadgoode and the stories she tells, is blasting through light-years of her own feminine emancipation. She enrolls in a course entitled "Assertiveness for Southern Women," (which she worries might be a contradiction in terms), greets her husband at the door of her house wrapped in cellophane, tears down walls in her suburban home with a sledgehammer, joins a fitness club, and takes a job as a Mary Kay sales rep. Her fragrances would have evolved as well, and she would have found new inspiration in one of her "own" Mary Kay fragrances, particularly *Angelfire,* a floral woody musk fragrance launched in 1977.

Inspired indeed. Evelyn was surely fired by some combination of fragrances and Idgie's stories when she finally let loose in the parking lot of a Winn Dixie grocery store. Her cool response to the incredulous victims of her outrage tells everything about the confidence a fragrance can give a woman, whatever her situation in life.

Moral: Whether practicing grand larceny, revenge, or petty thievery, don't forget your perfume, and remember to share the inspiration of your stories and fragrances with your Bad Girl friends. Tawanda!

◈

◈ CHAPTER FIVE ◈

The Huntress

For millions of years, Bad Girl Huntresses have been roaming the forests and savannas of the planet finding and getting whatever in the world they want. No wonder they're so adept at hunting. Over countless millennia, hunting has become an integral part of Bad Girls' DNA. Indeed, after seduction, hunting is the oldest and most developed of all Bad Girl techniques, and Bad Girl Huntresses, like their seductress sisters, know the importance of perfumes tailor-made to their needs and desires.

Luckily, even after factoring in development from rural to urban environments, basic hunting techniques have remained the same throughout the centuries. The primary differences between modern Bad Girls hunting and traditional Bad Girl hunting are, 1.) The "chase" has become as much fun as the capture, and 2.) (In most cases, at least) Bad Girls want to stun, not kill, their prey.

Although there's no such thing as a "Perfume Hunting License," if you think of perfume as being (metaphorically) at least as powerful as a loaded gun, you can understand the importance of knowing how to use it correctly.

Whether for urban or rural environments, all Bad Girl

Huntress perfumes need to be properly calibrated, and offer some kind of camouflage or "silencer effect" to blend with the background and/or soften the impact. You don't want to haul out the perfume equivalent of a rifle or a bazooka if what you need is a pistol. And you certainly don't want the loud crack of a perfumed pistol shot if you're hunting in the quiet of the forest. Thus fragrances with soft green aromatic, woody, or leather notes, are particularly popular with ace Bad Girls Huntresses.

* Diane de Poitiers – Renaissance Bad Girl Huntress *Par Excellence*

As the mistress of King Henri II of France, (and therefore the hated rival of Henri's *wife* and Queen of France, the Florentine princess, Catherine de Medici), Diane de Poitiers (1499-1566) was obliged to deploy countless skills to maintain her position as Henri's mistress in the dangerous machinations and political intrigues of the court.

The French, not being as advanced in the ways of perfumery as the Florentine Italians at the time, Diane, though a reputed Renaissance beauty, had to contend with the more sophisticated perfume power of Catherine de Medici (as we shall see in greater detail in *Chapter 9: Cool Under Fire*.)

Playing decisively in Diane's favor, however, was her lover's passion for hunting sports and the fact that she, herself, was an ace Bad Girl Huntress. Indeed, so aligned was Diane in spirit with the huntress of mythology, the Roman Goddess Diane (Greek Goddess Artemis), that she adopted the Goddess's crescent moon as her emblem.

Thus, by calling on the advantages of her own superior hunting skills (as a Florentine, Catherine de Medici was more of a "city-state" girl), and using a crafty mixture of well chosen "Made in France" Bad Girl Huntress fragrant products Diane was able keep the heart of her lover all the way to the end of his life.

As a fine lady of the Renaissance, Diane would have perfumed her elegant hunting clothing with fragrant herbs (basil, chamomile, lavender, or thyme). On her person, she might have applied a form of toilet water dating from the 14th century, known as *Eau de la Reine de Hongrie,* composed of alcohol and rosemary and reputed for its health and beauty benefits. (More on this in Chapter 9: Cool Under Fire.) In the evening, after the exhilaration of the chase, she and her lover would have retired to the comforting fragrances of her chateau, adorned with dried juniper, briar, pine branches, or the leaves and stems of Sweet Flag (Acorus Calamus) which release a refreshing lemony scent when crushed.

Modern Bad Girl Huntresses and moon mistresses have many more fragrances at their disposition. I can imagine a fiery young and independent huntress like Diane, riding to hounds with her merry band of maids, wearing Charna Ethier's all natural *Moss Gown,* complex and soft as velvet. Confident and sophisticated, she's surrounded by familiar scents of the forest and revels in green and spirited *Amazone,* whose tartness reflects the black current buds growing along the paths. More mature Huntresses, at the height of their power, might imagine themselves like Diane and Henri in the full bloom of love, enjoying a quiet canter amid the green and woody notes of Maurer & Wirtz's warm and sensuous *Nonchalance,* or through the woods and valleys surrounding Chenonceau, the most romantic of Renaissance chateaux, and a gift from Henri to Diane. Henri would be wearing Hermès's quietly bold and woody fragrance *Terre d'Hermès,* that speaks of territory, earth, and roots.

Meanwhile, around the world and every day, lusty Bad Girl Huntresses happily drive their paramour foxes to ground accompanied by Jardin d'Ecrivain's woody and spicy fragrance, *Orlando,* while others bag their prey in The Vagabond Prince's *Enchanted Forest* surrounded by seductive glades of hawthorn, black current, balsam, and cedar. Still others prefer to silently lie in wait on early winter mornings while they breathe in the quiet presence of animals in the forest, surrounded by the soft mysteries of Parfums Volnay's *Brume d'Hiver.*

Pleasantly tired at the end of the day, and wrapped in the soft folds of Donna Karen's *Cashmere Mist,* they relax before a fire while savoring the warm leather and tobacco aromas of NICOLAÏ's *Vie de Château Intense.*

* Out of Africa – A Most Solitary Bad Girl Huntress

A very different early Twentieth Century Bad Girl Huntress graces Sydney Pollack's epic romantic drama, *Out of Africa,* in the character of the wealthy Danish woman, Karen Dinesen, AKA Isak Dinesen, (played by Meryl Streep). Having entered a marriage of convenience with her friend Baron Bror Blixen, in what she hoped would be a stable relationship lived out on a dairy farm, Karen finds herself with a philandering husband, a coffee plantation in Kenya, and immense solitude. Paradoxically, it is here that her life is exquisitely transformed by the wild beauty of the land, her deepest longings, and, of course, the power of perfumes. We, her husband, and her dinner guests get hints of this transformation well before she does, as the stories she tells of an evening reveal another Karen–a passionate adventuress. A solitary Bad Girl Huntress.

What was this call that she heeded, most unwillingly at times? Something stronger than her expectations and her will; some primal energy that spoke in dry *animalic* savanna fragrance tones of land, and fresh sensations of rain on green shoots of coffee plants; some carnal and overpowering desire for a fiercely independent man-lover, whom no woman could own.

As an aristocratic Danish woman of her time, Karen would have brought an array of perfumes with her to Kenya. Indeed, a surprising assortment of French, English, Italian, and German fragrances would have made their way with her by steamer and by rail over water and desolate lands to find their places on her spare and well-kept dresser. Their names like the liquids they contained, and the stories Karen would tell, were alliterative, and things of beauty in themselves: *L'Origan* by Coty, *Le Trèfle Incarnat* by L. T. Piver, *Vera Violetta* by Roger & Gallet, *Après l'Ondée* and *L'Heure Bleue* by Guerlain, *Violette Pourpre* by Houbigant, *La Rose d'Orsay* by D'Orsay, *Quelques Fleurs L'Original* by Houbigant, *Un Air Embaumé* by Rigaud, *Edwardian Bouquet* by Floris, *Bois de Cedrat* by Creed, *English Lavender* by Yardley, *Uralt Lavendel* by Lohse (now L'Oréal).

By day under the harsh glare of an equatorial sun, they would have mingled in the perspiration of her skin with the myriad fragrances of loud and lush native flowers, aromatic herbs and grasses. In the evening, they would have quieted her thoughts along with the aroma of bees wax tapers and kerosene lanterns. By night, they would have haunted her solitary dreams, or clashed and coupled like wild beasts with compelling yet elusive man odors and colognes – *Jean-Marie Farina, 4711,* or *Acqua di Biella N°1.*

As her only constant and intimate companions, her fragrances would have accompanied and encouraged her as she found her path through a world war, the free wildness of colonial East Africa, and the pervasive doubts that inevitably populate uncharted territories. Reluctantly but unquestionably, Karen would become of necessity, as courageous and romantic a Bad Girl Huntress as the heroines of her own stories. Ultimately, through the edition of her autobiographical writings, Karen would forever stalk the biggest game of all – the human heart.

Contemporary Bad Girl Huntresses of similar ilk would be well advised to stalk the plains and forests of eBay for Ralph Lauren's now, sadly, discontinued *Safari.* A dry and crisp, easily wearable green floral chypre crouching on a bed of dry woods, *Safari* was created by one of the world's greatest contemporary perfumers, Dominique Ropion. Meanwhile, huntresses dreaming of the woody coffee fragrances of exotic plantations should try Comme des Garçons *Series 7 Sweet: Wood Coffee.*

Nocturnal Huntresses will find light and rare shimmering beauty in Aedes de Venustas's soon to be released fragrance *Cierge de Lune,* based on the elusive and ethereal notes of the night-blooming cereus plant.

◈

◈ CHAPTER SIX ◈

Advanced Techniques for Special Prey

Having mastered perfume use for general hunting excursions, Bad Girls are quick to realize the importance of specific perfumes for special prey. Cougars, Gold Diggers, Mermaids, and Witches, listen up. Bad Girls Perfume is on your game.

* The Cougar

Urban legend has it that the term, "Cougar," referring to an older woman dating a younger man, was first coined in Canada during the 1980s to designate female fans of the *Canucks de Vancouver* ice hockey team who were older than the players they idolized. Now, of course, everybody on the planet knows that "Cougars" have been stalking younger prey since the beginning of time, some unsung and anonymous, others notoriously successful, and others still, infamous failures.

Out of respect for her talent, class, and sophisticated taste in perfume, I'm dedicating this chapter to a famous Cougar *failure.* "Here's to *you,* Mrs. Robinson!" And I mean it. What a gutsy woman you were in 1967. You, with your *chutzpa* and verve, ahead of your times sophistication, drop-dead *hottie* body, animal magnetism, jungle underwear, and there can be no doubt, great taste in perfume! I can imagine that when you met Benjamin for a "drink" at the Taft Hotel, you were wearing Carven's sultry chypre fragrance *Ma Griffe,* whose name in French means both "signature" and "claw." What, my dear woman, went wrong with your schemes? It couldn't have been your perfume, so I'm guessing it was simply a matter of poor timing.

Hey, wait a minute, I hear my readers saying. This woman was an aggressive, predatory harpy, who cheated on her husband, seduced a kid half her age, didn't hesitate to undermine her own daughter's happiness, and took to the bottle.

OK. OK. I hear you.

All I'm saying is that Mrs. Robinson was an exemplar Cougar in all ways but one: her exit strategy was pitiful. Primarily, I believe, because as an unhappily married middle-aged woman in the 1960s, her options were limited, so like many others of her generation, she took her exit down the slippery slide of alcoholism. If she'd been operating in during just about any other decade, her Cougar game would have surely flourished. (Take a moment to thank your 1968 sisters, Bad Girls. Without them your lives might have been as bleak as hers!)

By today's standards, for example, the forty-year old Mrs. Robinson would be considered a "kid," barely old enough to even be considered a "Cougar," and, frankly, a *hottie.* God knows what she might have done. First of all, she would *never* have been forced to give up her artistic career (or any career), to become financially dependent on a man she didn't love simply because she had his baby. She'd have organized some kind of day care, and opened a gallery, become the creative director of an edgy fashion brand, or editor of a trendy women's magazine. Hey, we all know this is a juggling act, but Mrs.

Robinson would have managed just fine. Furthermore, if, in the craziest of circumstances, she'd somehow met up with the likes of Benjamin, she would have ditched him *real fast,* once she caught wind of just how totally neurotic and mixed up he was, not to mention his most complicated romantic situation. Bye-Bye, Benjy! In two clicks of a mouse pad, she would have logged back on to tinder.com, and within a few hours would have been happily sipping martinis with any of a slew of young men, or several at a time (heck, we're not Bad Girls for nothing!) and charging it all to her expense account.

So, before you turn the page on Mrs. Robinson, let me give you a little assignment. First, watch *The Graduate* again. A great film in its time, it's even better today. Mrs. Robinson is 40 years old in the film, and Anne Bancroft who played the role was 36 at the time of filming.

After completing this part of the assignment, check your own driver's license, girlfriend, do the math, look in the mirror, and reflect on this: In 1967, the time of *The Graduate,* forty was considered "over-the-hill." There was even a popular expression among college students at the time, "Never trust anyone over thirty!" Today, millions of women, at least Mrs. Robinson's age, *and their lovers,* would disagree with this statement.

For all you Bad Girl Contemporary Cougars getting ready to go out on a prowl tonight, I suggest that you consider the powers of some highly effective floral chypre fragrances such as Vivienne Westwood's luscious and sparkly *Libertine,* Frédéric Malle's warm and spicy *Portrait of a Lady,* or Majda Bekkali darkly imbalanced *Tendre Est La Nuit* (Tender Is The Night).

Meanwhile, for the Bad Girl Cougar secure enough to flaunt, not hide, the *ripeness* of her flesh, I recommend Etat Libre d'Orange's leather chypre, *Charogne* (which means 'carrion' in French), while the most self-satisfied cougar of them all will find herself true personality reflected in Olfactive Studio's chypre fragrance, *Selfie.*

To borrow the words from another great 60s hit song, "The times they are a changing!"

* The Gold Digger

No one in recorded history has outdone Cleopatra (Cleopatra VII Philopator, 69-30 BC) as a Bad Girl Gold Digger in the success of her colossal ambitions and schemes. Not once, but twice did this girl *successfully* set her mind on the golden power and glory of the Roman Empire.

Highly cultivated, Cleopatra was well versed in the power of perfume and didn't hesitate to deploy it along with her other considerable *means* to accomplish her objectives. It is said she even perfumed the sails of her boats!

In 48 BC, a 22-year old Cleopatra had herself smuggled to Caesar rolled in a Persian rug. Prior to submitting to this steamy "wrap," and to ensure a totally sensual fragrance delivery, Cleopatra would have certainly bathed in a sophisticated blend of warm and fragrant floral, woody, and spicy Egyptian oils. A contemporary Cleopatra could obtain similar results by bathing in Estée Lauder's "In Your Face" warm and spicy oriental fragrance *Youth Dew.*

Interestingly, just as Cleopatra successfully slipped past her brother's guards wrapped in a carpet, *Youth Dew,* launched in 1953, slipped past an unspoken taboo of the 1950s that women of refinement received, but did not purchase, perfumes for themselves. Nothing was written about purchasing "bath oils" though, so by cleverly marketing *Youth Dew* as a "bath oil" and not a "perfume," Estée Lauder, like Cleopatra, found her way to her audience, fortune, and fame.

Mission accomplished, our Bad Girl Cleopatra enjoyed several years of power and wealth as the consort of a smitten Caesar until his unfortunate assassination in 44 BC.

Newly in need of Roman "gold," Cleopatra set her sights on Marc Antony who now governed the Roman Empire's eastern region, which included the kingdom of Egypt. So magnificent was Cleopatra's 41 BC journey to meet Marc Antony in Tarsus, and so blatant her use of fragrances, that it was recorded by the celebrated Roman historian, Plutarch. He describes her as arriving on a barge scented with exotic perfumes, reclining on deck in trappings of gold and jewels, and surrounded by thousands of flowers. Another legendary Bad Girls Perfume success.

Cleopatra's sizzling affairs with Caesar and Marc Antony burst to 20th Century (Fox) life in the 1963 Academy Award-winning film, *Cleopatra,* starring Elizabeth Taylor, Rex Harrison (Caesar) and Richard Burton (Marc Antony). Bringing her own Bad Girl magnetism and temperament to the role, Taylor more than fleshed out the life and character of Cleopatra. Indeed, the scandalous and steamy *life imitating art* Taylor-Burton love affair that erupted on set and in the tabloids during the movie's filming only added Technicolor proportions and juicy 20th century gossip to Cleopatra's legend.

Cleopatra, was as skilled in perfumery as any Bad Girl in history, and in many ways helped write the Bad Girls Perfume book. I've put her in this chapter because examples of her exploits in this category are the best documented, but in addition to excelling as a Gold Digger, it goes without saying that she was a Seductress. Additionally she knew how to work both Undercover and "In Your Face," was adept as

Bad Girl Sorceress, and, when necessary, never shrank from Making War, not Love.

Contemporary Cleopatras of similar Gold Digging disposition will surely find resonance in Elizabeth Taylor's own fragrance, *White Diamonds,* an "In Your Face" white floral, launched in 1987. An immediate "best-seller," *White Diamonds* was among the first of what would later be referred to as "celebrity" fragrances, and holds its own today, often ranked among the top 10 Christmas sellers.

More recently, an entire population of Bad Girl Gold Diggers swears by the age-old adage that the way to a man's heart is through his stomach, and depends on "gourmand" fragrances to get the job done. These girls claim that nothing is more appetizing for a gentlemen of means than a fresh and saucy Bad Girl *babe* served up in tasty layers of mouth watering, fruity, cotton-candy, or chocolate gourmand fragrance notes. The cult favorite of these Bad Girl Gold Diggers is Thierry Mugler's *Angel.* As the first "gourmand" fragrance, created in 1992, *Angel* was both ground breaking and earth shaking in its now iconic blue star-shaped and refillable bottle. Many users claim that *Angel* is impossible to resist, and a few go as far as to say it's addictive. In any event, no one has requested a "low calorie" version of this oriental vanilla seductress, and rumor has it that even more Mugler gourmandize is on the way in 2016....

Other gourmand favorites high on the list for Bad Girl Gold Diggers are the high-calorie and elegant vanilla and caramel treat, *Prada Candy,* the discerning vanilla and raspberry notes of *Passion de l'Amour* by House Of Sillage, the apple, cinnamon and coconut, *La Danza della Libellule* (dance of the dragonflies) by Nobile 1942, and the classy, more subtle, but equally nourishing *Dolce Riso* (Sweet Rice) by Calé Fragranze d'Autore.

Bad Girl Gold Diggers going after golden boy gourmands tending to lighter fare, know that Hermès sophisticated and minimalist *Un Jardin Sur le Nil,* with its delicate green mango peel and carrot notes, offers a fresh and equally enticing dessert alternative.

And if the quarry happens to be a highly cultivated connoisseur of wines and foods, along with the good and high Continental life, Gold Diggers can impress him with a taste of Rubini Profumi *Fundamental,* a complex fragrance with crisp and fruity, absolutely full-bodied aromatic grape notes. Definitely a grand cru!

Gold diggers with artistic leanings and a feminist bent can attract gourmand connoisseurs of the arts and fine alcohols with Arquiste for J.Crew's warm and sophisticated fragrances, *N°57* and *N°31.* The names of the fragrances are derived from their inspiration – aromas of the perfumes, cocktails, and warm woods surrounding the crowd at the *vernissage* of the first all-woman modern art show of the 20th Century, *Exhibition by 31 Women,* presented by Peggy Guggenheim in January, 1943 at The Art of This Century Gallery on New York's 57th Street. *Pour la petite histoire,* there were plenty of Bad Girls circulating at the show wearing a number of Bad Girls perfumes, notably Frida Kahlo, one of the artists in the exhibition, who was purportedly wearing Elsa Schiaparelli's 1937 fragrance, *Shocking.*

On another register, bright and inspirational Bad Girl Gold Diggers eager to lure aging millionaires with hopes of fresh new life, count on Britney Spears' fruity chypre fragrance *Believe,* while those eager to sooth a fabulously rich Prince Charming turn on their own charm with the softly feminine, clean and caressing *Swan Princess* by The Vagabond Prince. The gentle caresses of Marc Jacobs' youthful and pert *Daisy* promise soft summer afternoons lolling in field of flowers, while Lolita Lempicka's fresh and green *Lolita Lempicka* brings classic sophistication to the age old formula of eternal rejuvenation.

The youngest, most badass *rocker* of Bad Girl Gold Diggers can entice the wealthiest and most sentimental of *BoBo* Boomers with Room 1015's *Power Ballad* and its references to rebellious high school days of stressed leather, liquor, chewing gum, and French kisses. With a little luck her *BoBo* Boomer might even have been present during the mythical and decadent summer of 1972 when, among other things, Rolling Stones guitarist Keith Richards threw a television set out the window of room 1015 of LA's Sunset Strip Continental Hyatt House Hotel. Wild and riotous debauchery guaranteed.

The liveliest Bad Girl Gold Diggers play for hours with Yves Saint Laurent's laughing and seductive *Baby Doll,* while others prefer to simply taunt their lovers with Paris Hilton's "In Your Face" *Tease.* Meanwhile, over-the-top "Energizer Bunny" Bad Girl Gold Diggers can turn on the power (hopefully being careful not to wear these poor guys out) with the spicy accords of *Miss Wild* by Joop!.

* The Mermaid

From time immemorial, Bad Girl Mermaids have been calling men away from firm footing on land to deep water, hidden shoals, or ever-receding horizons. Early mermaid legends date as far back as 1000 BC in what is now Syria, but the most enduring myth in our time comes from the "Syrenes" or "Sirens" in Homer's *Odyssey.* In Greek mythology, sirens were creatures with voices of angels, upper bodies of beautiful women, and the cold hearts of man-eating, fishlike predators. They sat on rocks and shores and sang so seductively and compellingly that anyone who heard them was so possessed that they rushed to certain doom. Homer's hero, Odysseus (Ulysses in Latin), knew something about the irresistible call of Mermaids. Enough to order his men to lash him to the mast of his ship as he approached their islands. Even so, upon hearing them he did go mad with desire and begged his men to unbind him. It was to no avail since he had also ordered his men to plug their ears with wax.

Ah yes, much has been written about the *songs* of Mermaids. Yet I'm here to tell you that Mermaids' *real* power is in their fragrance. Homer, of course, omitted any details of mermaid fragrances in his tales, but it doesn't take much imagination to know they would smell like some combination of the tropical flowers they wore in their hair, the fruits and coconuts that grew on their islands, and the bracing ozone-y air of breaking waves. Most importantly, however, the most fascinating and alluring thing about a mermaid is the animalic, *female* odor of her tail. Without her tail or the odor of her tail, the mermaid loses at least half her power, as we shall see.

In contrast to Homer's Mermaids who were clearly and powerfully predatory, the mermaid in Hans Christian Andersen's 1837 tale, *The Little Mermaid* is portrayed as being innocent, sweet, and sometimes even helpful toward men. I don't buy this Mermaid "good intentions" interpretation for one minute. For one thing, anyone with even a cursory understanding of mermaid physiology is going to know her intentions would have to be "conflicted" at best, which definitely qualifies her as a Bad Girl. The way I see it, we never get a chance to see the true intentions of Andersen's little mermaid simply because once on dry land she has no power to carry them out. You'll remember that before she came ashore as a woman, she traded her fragrant mermaid tail for the much longed for legs of a human. Indeed, without the fragrance of her tail, Andersen's "sweet" little Mermaid finds that her powers of seduction are considerably diminished, and she ultimately loses all to the treachery of a man guided by human laws.

The moral to this Mermaid's *tale* lies in the Mermaid's *tail.* When venturing onto the shores of man, a well-advised Bad Girl Mermaid should never leave her tail – or at least the fragrance of her tail – behind.

Modern perfumery to the rescue. Taking cues from mermaid history, numerous perfume brands have rallied to the Bad Girl Mermaid's cause by concocting an abundance of quite effective fragrances to help them achieve their ends.

Starting in 1927, Jean Patou created *Huile de Chaldée,* the first commercial perfumed suntan oil (AKA Bad Girl Mermaid tail fragrance). Patou loaded *Huile de Chaldée* with hot sultry mermaid fragrances such as tropical florals, vanilla, and amber. What's more, *Huile de Chaldée's* mermaid tail fragrance was both "In Your Face" and ALL OVER YOUR BODY. A single whiff conjured an abundance of tanned, oiled, fragrant, and glowing flesh, beaded with droplets of salt water, exposed in the skimpiest of attire against the most primal of backdrops – sun, sand, and surf.

Needless to say, Patou's *Huile de Chaldée* was enormously successful. Recognizing a huge and hungry market for the unique powers of his fragrance, Patou created a perfume called simply *Chaldée* using the same notes as *Huile de Chaldée.*

Huile de Chaldée inspired the creation of many other suntan oil companies, and variations on Patou's fragrance formula become the signature of marine and beach fragrances for years to come. In France, the best-known brand to follow the sun after *Huile de Chaldée* was L'Oréal's *Ambre Solaire* in 1935, (now sold under the brand name, Garnier), which like *Huile de Chaldée* oozed with the aroma of tropical flowers. Across the Atlantic, *Coppertone* captured the coconutty appeal of tropical paradises. Other important North American brands included *Bain de Soleil* and *Ski and Ski.*

But it didn't stop here. Following Patou's lead, many fragrance companies simply bypassed the suntan lotion aspect of the product, and created (alcohol-based) perfumes that mimic the sensual notes of suntan oils. *Eau des Merveilles* by Hermès, for example, echoes the warm and sultry notes of Patou's *Huile de Chaldée,* Bond No.9's *Fire Island* captures *Ambre Solaire' s* enthralling smell of warm skin on hot sand, while Estée Lauder's *Bronze Goddess* and Guerlain's *Lys Soleia* recall the sultry notes of *Bain de Soleil.*

In the 1980s and 90s, a parallel strand of marine or "aquatic" fragrances emerged from the tides following the availability of calone, a synthetic raw material with an ethereal, ozon-y smell, evoking sensations of breaking waves, sea-breezes, and marine life.

Meanwhile, the brand, Carthusia, from the Island of Capri, claims that the recipe for its fragrance, *Ligea la Sirena,* named after Ligea, one of the very Mermaids who charmed Homer's Odysseus, was handed down from local monks who knew her. To understand why *Ligea la Sirena* might be a close interpretation of her fragrance, just imagine these poor innocent monks doing their damndest to live peacefully on the Island of Capri and focus on their "good" works, with the songs and swishing tails of Mermaids all about them. Reading between the lines of the Carthusia brand's history, it's easy to understand what these monks were really up to while coming up with the original formula for this feminine and sensual, sweet, honey-like fragrance.

Today, Bad Girl Mermaids have access to hundreds of beach and aquatic mermaid fragrances, and though often drenched in sunshine or the ozone-y energy of a bracing ocean breeze, they also carry a warning in their angelic harmonies: obsessive longings for the unfulfilled and that which can never be – an impossible union; an endless summer.

Needless to say, fragrances so powerful that they are simultaneously dangerous and compelling are basic equipment for Bad Girl Mermaids.

Imagine, for a moment how the story of Hans Christian Andersen's Little Mermaid might be different if she were to come ashore today. In this case, the "innocent" little mermaid would be able to deploy the full power of mermaid fragrances, and her Bad Girl Mermaid intentions would be clearly evident. Assuming she's a local girl, she might choose Zarkoperfume's *e'L* a mermaid fragrance native to Denmark with sensual floral green ozone-y sea notes. If, on the other hand, she has swum over from neighboring Ireland, she would surely wear Fragrances of Ireland's *Inis,* which means "the Energy of the Sea." The way Bad Girl Mermaids get around these days, she might even come from further afield in which case she might well wear Givenchy's *Fleur d'Interdit,* a floral, green, ozon-y, and aquatic suntan fragrance, Calvin Klein's romantic and feminine *Escape* with its hint of marine breezes, or perhaps even Issey Myake's ozon-y and other worldly *L'Eau d'Issey.*

In any event, instead of pining away for the love of The Handsome Prince, she would be happily lounging on the beach in some of her favorite fragrances, while a much less cocky Prince would be fighting off her potential boy toy suitors with a stick.

More recently and across the sea in Brazil, "The Girl from Ipanema" a child of the 60s, would unquestionably have been deploying the powers of *Coppertone,* by far the suntan lotion (AKA mermaid tail fragrance) of choice for several decades worth of North and South American Bad Girl Mermaids. Though walking on tall and tan human legs, The Girl from Ipanema was clearly a Mermaid, and a very, very Bad Girl Mermaid, at that. Having most carelessly aroused the longings and desires of Brazilian musicians Antonio Carlos Jobim and Vinicius de Moraes through the irresistible sillage of her *Coppertone,* she went on to ignite those same longings and desires of every man on every beach – from here to eternity. Who among us, man or woman, has not been moved by The Girl from Ipanema? The unattainable beach girl. A walking, strolling Mermaid.

Contemporary Ipanema Bad Girls and their North American sisters can accomplish equally devastating results with fragrances such as, CB I Hate Perfume's *At the Beach,* a cult favorite among beach perfume enthusiasts, or Bobby Brown's *Beach,* which smells about as close to *Coppertone* as you can get.

Bad Girl Mermaids whose lure is more saline or ozone-y than sunny and sultry can find satisfaction in James Heeley's breezy and aquatic *Sel Marin* or The Different Company's *Sel de Vetiver,* a woody aromatic fragrance with sea salt notes.

Though not technically a Mermaid, I'd be remiss in my Bad Girl duties if I didn't mention Calypso, a wood nymph who inhabited the island Ogygia, (located between Italy and Sicily) where Odysseus claimed to have been shipwrecked (for seven years, no less!). Clearly, this wood nymph chick had gotten the memo about men of the human species, and mermaid or not, she knew that what these dudes want is *tail.* No problem. Instead of marine notes, Calypso obviously created a (clearly successful) wood nymph tail allure from the harsh green notes of island shrubs similar to those in Parfum d'Empire's *Corsica Furiosa* (The Fury of Corsica). *Pour la petite histoire,* the fragrance *Corsica Furiosa* won the 2015 French Fragrance Foundation Experts ("Fifi") Award for Best Niche Brand fragrance. Bad Girl Mermaids looking to seduce juries as well as epic heroes, heed my tale!

Ultimately, it's only in the 1989 Disney film *The Little Mermaid,* that the impossible mermaid-human union is actually fulfilled, and as by now you've surely realized, it's largely thanks to the little mermaid's fragrance. For those of you with any lingering doubts, watch *The Little Mermaid* again, carefully this time, and you'll recognize this film as nothing less than an allegorical testimony to the absolute power of perfume, and mermaid tail fragrances in particular. As you'll remember, much is made of the fact that Ariel can't win the Prince without her voice. Savvy Bad Girls, of course, recognize this as nothing but a ruse to fool the Evil Sea Witch. The truth is, Bad Girl or not, as a tail-less woman, Ariel simply could not do it without the help of her favorite mermaid fragrance. Having somehow lost it in the commotion of coming to shore, she manages to recover it in the violent climax at the end of the film. If you watch closely, you'll notice that at the moment Ariel's voice flies towards her, there's a simultaneous *tiny* spray of what might appear to be sea foam, but in truth, it's a bottle of Bad Girl mermaid perfume or suntan lotion that her mermaid sisters have tossed up to her from the depths in a last ditch effort to save her.

I'll leave it to you to figure out which fragrance it was. My die-hard Bad Girl Mermaid friends are convinced it has to have been *Huile de Chaldée, Ambre Solaire,* or *Coppertone.* Others think it was NICOLAÏ's *Musc Monoï* with its neroli, jasmine, and coconut notes. Still others are adamant that it was Comptoir Sud Pacifique's *Coco Extreme.* There are even those dreamers who insist it was Estée Lauder's *Beyond Paradise,* which offers nothing less than a tropical fantasy in a perfect world of optimism and wonder. Who knows? Thanks to the magic of perfume, it might well turn out to be the fragrance of *your* most obsessive Bad Girl Mermaid beach memories.

* The Bad Girl Witch and The Attractive Forces of Darkness.

If I only offer here a furtive peek at the power of Bad Girl Witches and their use of perfume, it's because this formidable mixture is too dangerous a phenomenon to risk closing up between the pages of a book. My intention is therefore, and with great respect and humility, to simply blow open a window on one of fragrance's elemental strengths: its power to evoke the dark side. Whether truly The Dark Side, as in "Evil" with a capital E, or simply the incandescent feminine face of power, which has historically been associated with evil in all its forms, there can be no doubt that a cunning and crafty mix of perfumery and witchcraft is as good as bad gets!

Given the documented dangers and inconveniences of openly practicing witchcraft, witnessed by the fact that throughout history witches have met with unhappy, often violent deaths, you don't need to have been turned into a frog yesterday to realize that the part of witchcraft typically identified with pointy hats, green faces, and ugly warts represents but a tiny tip of the witchcraft iceberg. So, while there are relatively few "In Your Face" Bad Girl Witches, you can be sure that myriads of Bad Girl Witches around the world practice witchcraft "undercover" on a daily and nightly basis, often ensconced in comfortable domesticity.

Samantha Stephens from the 1960s TV show *Bewitched* is an excellent case in point, with Samantha (played by Elizabeth Montgomery) disguised as a "normal" housewife. Little does her bumbling husband know that lurking behind his wife's Good Girl (though also alluring and feisty) persona is a bonefide Witch of considerable talents (except, perhaps in choosing a husband). At any moment, and in the name of carrying out her Bad Girl Witch-ly duties, she's ready to use her "Truth Spell" and other tricks, certainly including an array of funny, sneaky, and sexy fragrances she could easily levitate from the counters of her local department store. I imagine that she surely casts many a spell with Le Galion's *Sortilège,* with its refined and elegant rose, lily, and jasmine opening and its *animalic* Bad Girl dry-down. And when all she needs to do is totally distract her husband, a single well-placed drop of Dana's *Tabu* works magic.

Meanwhile, in the 1987 American comedy-fantasy film, *The Witches of Eastwick,* based on John Updike's novel of the same name, three witches, though certainly not what anyone would call domesticated, attempt to discreetly blend in with the quaint, picturesque, and uber conservative New England town of Eastwick, Rhode Island. Things start getting complicated when they decide to set up housekeeping as a lovely little *ménage à quatre* (four). No that's not a typo. The three women, Alexandra, Jane, and Sukie, played respectively by Cher, Susan Sarandon, and Michelle Pfeiffer, are first seduced by, and then *share* one man, the self-described "horny little devil" Daryl Van Horne (brilliantly played by Jack Nicholson). Not to worry, girls, there's plenty of what this guy's got to go around! For one thing (although this seems to have been censored from the film), he's wearing one hell of a satanic fragrance concoction, and I'm guessing it's Nu Be's *Sulphur [16S]*. Indeed, in the end, Van Horne turns out to be more than a handful, all of which leads to a wild adventure of sex and magic.

Ironically, it's only when Van Horne betrays the women, that they discover their real powers (sound familiar?) and the rest of the film ignites in hilarious "In Your Face" Bad Girl Witch revenge antics. Though also apparently censured from the script, it's not hard to imagine the explosive alchemy of three outstandingly wicked perfumes that appeared as if by magic during the decade preceding the film. Lancôme's 1978 *Magie Noire* is dark and barbaric as the three women realize the power they have to conjure revenge techniques, Calvin Klein's 1985 *Obsession* is wild and spicy as they begin to fire each other up for carrying out their revenge, and Dior's 1985 *Poison* proves its noxious effects as the women's magical works begin to show.

Driven mad by their powers, a totally deranged Van Horne curses God and rants, "Women! Is it a mistake? Or did he do it to us on purpose?" Oooooh! How gloriously wicked. Eve would be so proud.

Twenty years later, in the multi-season TV series *Charmed,* three sisters, Piper, Phoebie, and Page don't hesitate to use an array of Bad Girl Witch tricks and devices, even after discovering that they are the most powerful *good* witches in the world. Storming around in spike heels and other trappings of Bad Girls power, its clear that these "Charmed Ones" as they are called, are also making good use of the excellent Bad Girls perfumes which magically materialized around the time of the series. To help fight evil while maintaining impeccable disguises as everyday (albeit classy and sexy) good girls, our heroines are undoubtedly utilizing CHANEL's rich and complex *Allure* (1996), and Dior's luminous and opulent *J'Adore* (1999) to manage this aspect of the job with verve and class. Meanwhile, conjuring such dark powers as freezing time, is easily accomplished with Céline's 1966 bewitching and spicy *Magic,* predicting and rearranging the future is a cinch with Estée Lauder's warm and golden *Intuition,* while Liz Claiborne's opulent floral bouquet *Curve* (1996) is perfect for the job of causing objects and people to move against their will, and proves versatile enough for home and office use.

Doing all this in the name of "getting the job done," of course, places these "Charmed Ones" squarely in the middle of the Bad Girl Witches category (and first rate, at that), all of which can perhaps best be summed up in Chopard's (2001) sharp and volatile fragrance, *Madness.*

Today's "Charmed Ones" would lead the way among contemporary Bad Girl witches in wearing and honoring *Opus 1144,* Unum's warm and shadowy fragrance bearing the magic numbers associated with the official birth of Gothic in Europe. Whether depending upon daily incantations of the sensual musks in Rouge Bunny Rouge's *Incognito* or the stunning powers of X-Ray's *Morphine* to triumph over the forces of Evil, they would continuously bolster and purify their spirits with Diane Pernet's protective fragrance, *In Pursuit of Magic.*

Meanwhile, late in the 20th century a witch of a completely different profile emerged from the Harry Potter fantasy novels and films. Thanks to unprecedented historical and social changes, the young Hermione Granger (Emma Watson) manages to practice "In Your Face" witchcraft and still be enormously attractive to guys. In fact, Hermione's skills in witchcraft are in large part what win the approval and affection of none other than Harry Potter, himself (Daniel Radcliffe), and Ron Weasley (Rupert Grint), leading to what might easily be interpreted as a *ménage à trois.* Oh, la-la! Could our most virtuous Hermione Granger, heroine of the Harry Potter series, be a Bad Girl?

Although initially appearing bookish and rule-bound, Hermione reveals her free Bad Girl Witch spirit early in the first term at Hogwarts School of Witchcraft and Wizardry when in addition to learning magic, she doesn't hesitate to break all sorts of rules including, but not limited to, trespassing, breaking the laws of time travel, making up stories, lying, blackmail, and memory modification.

We even get an early hint of the types of Bad Girls fragrances Hermione might have been carrying in her "charmed handbag," along with her wand and "Time-Turner" when she smells freshly mowed grass and new parchment in "The Love Potion" (which supposed smells different for people according to what attracts them). Turns out that these are scents she associates with Ron, the love of her life. Two fragrances come to mind, both of which contain the synthetic molecule, coumarin, which in perfumery adds a sweetish note similar to that of mown hay or freshly cut grass. These are Floris's fresh and young, slightly tart green floral fragrance, *Florissa,* and

Burberry's outrageous, always charming, and unpredictably sexy, *Burberry Brit.*

Other hints about Hermione's choice of fragrances can be found in the fact that two plants are commonly associated with some of her favorite spells and potions: the Mandrake root, a Eurasian plant with purple flowers and a forked root, and Bluebells, native to England. From this it's easy to deduce that Hermione might wear Annick Goutal's fragrance *Mandragore,* which contains the Mandrake root. Chances are also strong that she might choose Penhaligon's beguiling green floral fragrance, *Bluebell,* or Jo Malone's linear and naughty, *Wild Bluebell.*

Meanwhile, having surely heard tales that many talented Bad Girl witches never return from its pleasures, Hermione would take great care when practicing "time travel" on the incense, woody, and leather notes of MiN New York's magical fragrance, *Forever Now.*

Maleficent, the 2014 Disney film, and the starring character, Maleficent, offer the perfect fairy tale Bad Girl Witch – a strong woman who truly enjoys being bad, while revealing the story behind the Sleeping Beauty fairy tale. Angelina Jolie brilliantly portrays this magnificent character. To refresh your memory, Maleficent ("Mistress of All Evil" in Disney's 1959 film *Sleeping Beauty*) first causes the princess Aurora to fall into a deathlike sleep by pricking her finger on a spindle, and then opposes The Prince who can supposedly break the spell with a kiss. There can be no mistake about Maleficent's evil. And yet, in the 2014 Disney film which reveals the truth of how the young Maleficent lost her fairy wings and goodness, Maleficent the woman, and her powers of witchcraft, *magically* become loveable and sexually appealing.

To augment her power and charms, the character Maleficent would certainly use perfumes and concoctions with dark hearts to be conjured by mysterious esoteric chants and phrases. Given her colossal task of personal transformation from the dark side to the light, she would be drawn to *Les Eaux-Delà* (a play on words that can be interpreted as "Fragrances of The After-life"). This first powerful and volatile fragrance trilogy from Philippe di Méo's brand Liquides Imaginaires, is rumored to possess cleansing and beneficial emotional and sacred properties. Maleficent would also love the wickedly expensive two-foot tall pewter *amphora* vessels designed to contain the fragrances. Each is engraved with cryptograms and symbols of sacred geometry. Luckily, for Bad Girl Witches of more modest means, the entire and much expanded Liquides Imaginaires fragrance line, though still otherworldly, also exists in 100 ml (3.38 oz.) bottles and even as candles, especially favorable for conjuring spirits.

Maleficent would also enjoy experimenting with her test tube of Zero Zero's *Blood Perfume* and its cold and clinical formula for raw sexual desire. She would also surely keep plenty of Il Profumo's *Black Dianthus* on hand with its black carnation note, an enigmatic magic potent both female on the skin and masculine in its heart, which the spirits say beats to the rhythms of the animals of the forest.

Meanwhile, for soothing her nerves while searching the clouds for hints of her future, Maleficent might use alternate doses of Ulrich Lang New York's patchouli and leather, soft and quietly dark *Nightscape,* Mark Buxton's *Emotional Rescue,* with its sharp and uplifting powers of vetiver, or Puredistance's *Black* whose warm and silky oud notes can transform the darkest of night into the softest of velvet.

Wood sprites inhabiting the forest around her castle have even reported that in playful moments, Maleficent gives in to the pleasures of her own dark humor, and spritzes herself with *Estratto di Follia* (Extract of Madness) by Peccato Originale (Original Sin), and that during "Happy Hour" she loves to chase her pet raven and sprinkle him with Frapin's dark and metallic, yet sharp and spicy fragrance, *Never More.*

For anyone wondering what makes a Bad Girl like Maleficent tick, an examination of her Map of the Heart fragrances offers a glimpse of the breath and complexity of the Bad Girl Witch perfume psyche – innocent *Rose Heart,* passionate *Red Heart,* dark *Black Heart,* noble *Gold Heart,* and valiant *Purple Heart.*

Ultimately, all Bad Girls, whether they consider themselves to be witches or not, are born with an innate predisposition for the techniques of witchcraft. And Savvy Bad Girls know you don't have to be a bonefide Witch with a capital 'W' (or 'B' as some like to think) to excel at this, as long as you use the most basic ingredient in all magic formulas: perfume.

An excellent example of a favorite every day, and relatively simple Bad Girl Witch trick is that of creating obsessive feelings of desire and longings by disappearing, or simply *appearing* to disappear. Among themselves, Bad Girls use the code "Smoke and Mirrors" to refer to this trick.

A champion in this most devastating art of sorcery, and the epitome of the "Smoke and Mirrors" Bad Girl is Maybellene, the iconic Bad Girl who inspired the 1955 Chuck Berry rock and roll hit, *Maybellene.* Though her true identity is never revealed in the song, I have it on the best authority that Maybellene is none other than the 17-year old Bad Girl daughter of a small town USA Cadillac dealer. Through the exhaust smoke and rear view mirror of her Cadillac *Coup de Ville,* we follow Maybellene in an ace Bad Girl "Smoke and Mirrors" driving demo of how a wicked combination of fragrance and makeup, Maybelline, of course, can be used for deception and amusement, all the while leading a hapless local swain on a merry game of chase.

Pour la petite histoire, the spelling of the girl's name in the song, Maybellene, was deliberately different from that of the makeup brand, Maybelline, in order to avoid a possible lawsuit.

My Bad Girl Witch friends and I agree that Maybellene's fragrance is, and forever will be, *Intimate,* the green chypre fragrance by Revlon, which like herself, was fresh out of the box in 1955. Meanwhile, her hit tune, *Maybellene,* will remain the song of choice for cruising urban and suburban Bad Girls, accompanied, of course, by indispensable makeup and fragrance refreshers, hastily applied while idling at red lights.

Still shrouded in mystery, we get another tantalizing glimpse of our "Smoke and Mirrors" champion in the 1973 George Lucas cult 60s film, *American Graffiti.* This time she's the disappearing blond driving a white '56 Ford T-Bird, just a hill-top, stop light, or payphone call ahead of her current (and still hapless) swain, Curt (Richard Dreyfuss). She is doubtless wearing Prince Matchabelli's warm and spicy *Wind Song,* created in 1953 and immensely popular throughout the 60s.

Eternally young, Maybellene was recently spotted on the same turf, burning up 21st century Bad Girl Witch macadam in a silver Lexus IS convertible. It's not Daddy's car though, it's hers. Daddy gave it to her on her 16th birthday as a reward for getting her driver's license the same day. More worldly than her 20th century "Smoke and Mirrors" predecessors, Maybellene has been around. The same summer of her

16th birthday, she visited her mom in Paris, and among other things, fell in love with the Marais. Those poor fellas back home! Still trying to find her, still desperately sifting through the smoke and mirrors of her fragrance clues, the most confusing of which exudes from the one she now keeps in her glove compartment: Comme des Garçons' *Garage.*

Though spending inordinate amounts of time passing on curves and speeding carelessly over the horizon along the wrong side of the yellow line, Maybellene and her Bad Girls Perfume Witchcraft astoundingly survives for eternity. We'll never see her face for more than an instant, but somewhere in her trail of exhaust smoke, misleading mirror images, discarded gum wrappers, and lingering fragrance notes of chypre, fruity florals, and synthetic kerosene, Maybellene, like a fleeting high school romance, will forever lure us over the edge and around one last curve towards excitement and unattainable longings.

◈ CHAPTER SEVEN ◈

Fantasies

Bad girls LIVE for fantasies. If you're like me, fantasies make up as much as 90% of your life. This being said, it's important to note that the most brilliant thing about fantasies is that the only "fact" about them is that nobody knows whether they're true or not. And this is great. Bad Girls need to keep people guessing and wondering. Would she *really* do that? To make it even more fun, even *we* don't know whether we will, or will not, act on our fantasies. Would *I* really do this? Does anybody even know I fantasize about that?

Fantasies open a fabulous secret world to hide from or run to, alone, or in company. Who or what could be our best accomplice for such exploits? Perfumes, of course. As keepers of the gates to our wildest, deepest, and most intimate imaginations, perfumes can inspire, encourage, and accompany us through all our fantasies, as we act, or don't act. And although the best perfumes leave an indelible "trail," they will never betray our deepest secrets. Unless, of course, we want them to.

So although nobody will ever catch *me* claiming these fantasies as my own, here are two of my favorites, *from the Street.* Recognize anybody around here? I won't tell.

* Messing Around with the Boss

Don't worry. I know you're not stupid. We all know you just *don't* mess around with the boss. This is rule number ONE in any career woman's book. I wouldn't do it. You certainly wouldn't do it. This is the kind of thing that can get you into way too much trouble. For sure. Never. Not even if.... No. NO. No no no no no no! Never means never! After all, you don't have to be born yesterday to know which side your bread is buttered on. So, forget it. No matter what. NO exceptions! Except of course.... As a matter of fact, now that you mention it, there was that time when.... And, oh yes, there was my good friend ___ ___, and she ended up....! But that was a special case. And, well anyway, I'm not going to tell you what to do. And of course, telling any Bad Girl about a rule is only going to excite her imagination, and telling her not to *break* a rule is just asking for trouble. So, forget it. No, don't forget it. Anyway, fair warning. And for the record, I did tell you not to do this. But just in case you have a friend or something, here's the story....

Two fragrances immediately come to mind for Bad Girls Boss fantasies: Etat Libre d'Orange's *Sécrétions Magnifiques* (Fabulous Secretions) and Thierry Mugler's *Womanity.* Both smell distinctly like – might as well man up to it – semen.

Sécrétions Magnifiques, like most Etat Libre d'Orange fragrances, was deliberately designed to be provocative and disturbing. Created in 2006 by Bad Boy perfumer Antoine Lie for Etat Libre d'Orange's equally Bad Boy founder, Etienne de Swardt, *Sécrétions Magnifiques* has doubtless generated as much hate mail as any scandalous and illicit office liaison ever did. There's no getting around it. *Sécrétions Magnifiques* smells like hot steamy sex. Its hard-hitting adrenalin punch ejects odors of all possible body liquids associated with sex:

blood, sweat, tears, semen, spit.... The works. Pervasive and tenacious, *Sécrétions Magnifiques* is also what is known as a "scrubber." Extremely hard to wash off. So, be careful how and when you use it, because no matter how doubtful the wisdom or future of whatever it is that you're up to, *Sécrétions Magnifiques* (which some people refuse to call a "fragrance"), leaves no doubt as to what it smells like. That's all there is to it.

Thierry Mugler's *Womanity,* on the other hand, is both sweet and savory, can smell like other things, and some people claim they don't notice the semen at all. Don't believe them. Anybody even *thinking* about messing around with the Boss is sure to claim or disclaim all sorts of stuff. Upon its creation in 2010, the Mugler team pushed the idea that *Womanity* was for women who wanted to feel "powerful and connected." OK. And I especially love the brand's seemingly innocuous description of *Womanity* as a "...casual perfume [that] has given women a distinctive way to express themselves, whether they are taking care of business or spending time with those they love." Hmmm....Whatever works. And just to drive home the point, the brand euphemistically refers to *Womanity's* signature tell-tale *animalic* note as a salty "caviar" note, and a "...rhythmic play between sweet and savory." In any event, thanks to other notes including citrus, fig, and woods, one has the feeling that the wearer is, at least, giving lip service to covering her trail, and might *just* get away with it. It's the kind of odor you've surely run across from time to time right after lunch when you've returned to your office ten minutes earlier than usual. Could be one of your Bad Girl co-workers (doubtless, a current reincarnation of *Mad Men's* Peggy Olson) started off the day wearing a fig or woody fragrance, and then just barely had time for a noon-time *quickie* before slipping –

oh, so smugly – back to her desk. Or maybe she just had time for a spurt of *Womanity.*

* Messing Around With the Hired Help

Ok, so imagine this…. You're in the kitchen and you've got this guy in there. He's either a plumber, electrician, painter, landscaper, or whatever. He's fixing something. And no matter where that something is, you can be sure that at some point he'll get in this *position* – don't know how they do it but they manage every time! He'll position himself with his head under the sink, and his jeans… (I'm sure these guys get them specially made for this. It's got to be a conspiracy.) Anyway, his jeans are half way down his butt. And he knows exactly what you're looking at. And he *knows* exactly what you're thinking. And he's right. You're thinking, 'Hmmmm. Nice ass!' And then you're thinking, 'What the hell should I do now? I already offered this dude a cup of coffee…and it's not like I can just go off and leave him here to his own devices in my house. 'Cause there's nobody else here. Won't be for at least a couple of hours. …. Not that he would steal anything. In fact, he seems like a nice guy. Cute, too. And friendly. Wonder if he's –? Didn't I see a little twinkle in his eye when he first walked in? Wonder what would happen if…. Na, that's ridiculous. Truly ridiculous. After all, I'm –! And he's surely –! And, anyway. Anyway, what–?' If any woman here tells me she hasn't had this fantasy, she's a liar!

Uniquely interesting about Hired Help Fantasies is that they typically come out of the blue and fly in the face of conflicting and negative emotions or prejudices, all of which create deliciously heightened tensions.

An excellent case in point is a Bad Girls fantasy that begins as a total blind-side and develops into a full-blown love story of continental proportions in the 2008 film *Australia*. At the beginning of the film, when Lady Sarah Ashley, (played by Nicole Kidman) flies from England to Australia she's thinking of one thing only, and that's to sell her husband's property there. It's 1939, and the last thing on her mind is a romantic interest, and certainly not with a filthy cattle drover from nowhere, and of doubtful pedigree. When forced to travel across the Outback with just such a grubby, albeit drop-dead sexy, cattle drover (played by Hugh Jackman) in the cramped quarters of a Land Rover, she hugs her side of the seat in an attempt to keep as far from him as possible. The only reason she even looks at him from beneath her prim hat and veil is to maintain a suspicious eye on the dreadful man. If you, the viewer, are able to look at anything *besides* Jackman, er I mean, Drover's chiseled and unshaven profile (which I doubt – I only forced myself to do so in order to research this piece), you will notice that Lady Sarah is clutching something to her chest. Turns out, that something is a handkerchief she's dabbed in fragrance in an attempt to protect herself from the stench. Little does she know, that her fragrance, Grossmith's *Hasu-no-Hana,* created in 1888 during a time of great pioneering spirit in perfumery, is also a Bad Girls fantasy perfume *par excellence,* and that instead of protecting her from this man, it's actually priming her for fantasy. Oh yes. Certain fragrances will do this, you know. After a day of unsuspecting fragrance priming by this bright and sensual floral chypre oriental fragrance, overflowing with the scent of the Japanese lotus lily, it doesn't take much to tip Lady Sarah irretrievably into fantasy. This, of course, happens that very evening when she is confronted with the sight of Drover's nude torso as he showers in the middle of the desert campground. I know, I know. Given the subject matter, she might well have entered into this fantasy without a drop of fragrance. The fantasy nature of *Hasu-no-Hana* only ensures that her fragrance fantasy will be so intense as to be totally irrevocable.

Unlike our Bad Girl friend in the kitchen whose fantasy has less than an hour to go real or not, Lady Sarah has the wide open spaces of Australia, unexpected complications, and the leisure of a feature length film to turn her Bad Girl perfume fantasy into a flesh and blood love affair. Given the size of her vanity case, she clearly has a well-stocked supply of her fantasy perfume, so wittingly or not, our heroic Lady Sarah is in no danger of running out of juice before the *fantastic* denouement.

Meanwhile, I can't abandon our contemporary Bad Girl in the kitchen. Even if faced with more prosaic prospects than those of Lady Sarah, I suggest she leave a bottle of Etat Libre d'Orange's *Fat Electrician* in a conspicuous place on the counter. Or, depending how things are progressing, instead of another cup of coffee she might offer to apply a little spritz. As for strategic locations, it's hard to beat Jane Avril's spot-on advice (in Chapter Two: The Two Faces of Eve) about where to apply a fragrance – mounds and crevasses. Chances are, she won't have to look far.

◈

◈ CHAPTER EIGHT ◈

When All Else Fails: Make War, Not Love

Women, unlike men, normally declare war only as a last resort, when all else has failed. If a woman declares war against a single individual, it's typically a former lover, from whom she can find no moral or physical escape, and war is an act of desperation. If on the other hand, she declares war on more than one person, more often than not, it's a former lover and rival duo, and her motivation is jealousy.

In either case, if war is inevitable, the right perfume is an essential ally. Before undertaking any such drastic actions Bad Girls might be well advised to check out a large volume of Jovoy's *L'Art de La Guerre* (The Art of Warfare), a bold feminine take on an otherwise leather and woody, manly fragrance. Anyone who gets to this point knows there can be no turning back.

In the 1965 film *Dr. Zhivago,* based on Boris Pasternak's 1957 novel, one of the moments of highest drama takes place at a Christmas Eve party when Lara Antipova (Julie Christie) shoots Victor Komarovsky (Rod Steiger) in an unsuccessful assassination attempt. The year is 1913, and the backdrop to both the book and the film is that of two historic wars – the Russian Revolution and the First World War. The central story though, is about doctor and poet/writer Yuri Zhivago (Omar Shariff), his love for Lara, and Lara's decades-long war of attrition with Komarovsky.

The shooting incident, Lara's initial declaration of war against Komarovsky, reveals Lara's rapidly evolving character as a courageous and inspiring Bad Girl, bravely navigating troubling times and the delicate shifting balance between her own dark and light sides. Although omitted from both the book and the film, there can be no doubt that just before thrusting the revolver into her muff and leaving home for the Christmas party, Lara would certainly have taken the time to hastily, yet *deliberately,* dab on Caron's *Narcisse Noir* (Black Narcissus). She would have done this because at some deep level she recognized *Narcisse Noir* as *her* perfume, and trusted its delicate balance of strength and frailty to embolden and accompany her in her resolve. In this defining Bad Girls Perfume moment, *Narcisse Noir* (created in 1911) is as revealing of Lara's character, as Maurice Jarre's much beloved musical score, *Lara's Theme.*

Memories of the subsequent events at the dazzling 1913 Christmas Eve party would forever be galvanized in the hearts and minds of the glittering Muscovite guests thanks to a unique combination and brutal confrontation of extraordinary fragrances. Floating around and above the crowd, a rich ether composed of aromatic pine resins from the enormous Christmas tree, beeswax candles, woody and metallic notes from polished parquet floors and gilded paneling, along with mellow tobacco notes from Cuban cigars. All this intermingled with a heady mixture of French, English, and Italian perfumes – Guerlain, Houbigant, Lubin, Grossmith, Yardley, Floris, Creed, Penhaligon's, Santa Maria Novella, Coty, L.T.

Piver – emanating from glowing and warm, silk, brocade, and kid clad bodies. This dreamlike ambiance was abruptly and irrevocably shattered by the sharp crack of a pistol shot, directly followed by a biting and hostile wind, swept into the ballroom by the sudden and unwelcome entrance of Pasha, Lara's fiancé and passionate revolutionary comrade, carrying with it acrid street smells of bonfires, unwashed skin and clothing, haggard and seething frustration, bitterness, and the specter of violent revolution.

Pour la petite histoire, Victor Komarovsky would *not* have been wearing *BRUT* Cologne by Faberge, although in name and composition this fragrance would have perfectly suited him. *BRUT* wasn't created until 60 years later in 1964, perhaps in "loving" memory of a man such as him. Instead, Komarovsky would most likely have been wearing a heavy-handed dose of the same fragrance he had worn for years, Houbigant's otherwise classy and classic, *Fougère Royale,* created in 1882 by Paul Parquet, and revolutionary at the time as the first "fougère" (fern-like) perfume. Upon the realization that Lara had shot him, Komarovsky collapsed in his chair and would have fainted, had not Dr. Prof. Boris Kurt, who happened to be standing nearby, discreetly administered a stiff dose of smelling salts. The resulting combined smell of ammonia, adrenalin, cold sweat, hot desire, and the lingering amber and woody base notes of *Fougère Royale,* would have contributed to the intensity of Yuri Zhivago's visceral dislike of Komarovsky, as he assumed the necessary medical duties of bandaging the (very slight) flesh wound.

For his part, Zhivago would have been wearing a classic Guerlain fragrance, *Mouchoir de Monsieur,* a secret gift his fiancée, Tonya, had brought back from her recent trip to Paris.

In doing so, Tonya had broken a cardinal rule of propriety (a well-bred woman in Imperial Russia would never have offered a fragrance to a man), and came as close as she ever would to being a Bad Girl. Tonya, in turn, would have been wearing François Coty's soft and romantic single floral fragrance, *La Rose Jacqueminot,* which she had purchased at Les Grands Magasins du Louvre while on the same trip to Paris. Indeed, it was on the floor of this fashionable department store, where only a few years earlier, in 1904, the young perfumer François Coty had dashed a bottle of *La Rose Jacqueminot,* his first perfume, when the perfume buyer had refused to place an order. According to legend, a crowd had immediately gathered, clamoring to buy the intriguing fragrance, thus marking the beginning of one of the most brilliant perfume careers in history.

Following his witnessing of the shooting and Lara's dramatic exit, Yuri Zhivago's body temperature would have surely risen intensely, causing the *Mouchoir de Monsieur* to evaporate, leaving only a dreamy iris and vanilla residue mixed with a not unpleasant smell of masculine body odor, and perhaps coloring his first inspirations to write the "Lara" poems. As for Lara's fiancé Pasha, he would have refused to wear any fragrance at all, cursorily dismissing it as an evil and corrupting "bourgeois affectation."

For the record: Following the failed assassination attempt, Lara's war with Komarovsky ultimately costs her the two great loves of her life, Zhivago, and her daughter by Zhivago. Even so, I would have changed nothing about Lara or her story – save one thing, and that *something* even the vast power of perfume couldn't do. I would have made her a better shot.

History has an uncanny way of repeating itself, and it's easy to imagine similar characters and their perfumes, if this drama were to erupt today at a holiday party in one of the world's glittering capitals. The lovely and conflicted Lara would vacillate between two fragrances, all the while continuing to inspire extraordinary emotions in every man she met. On some days she would wear Lancôme's soft and intoxicating fragrance, *Poême,* with its alliterative contrasts of bitter and sweet, while on other days, she would choose Miller Harris's *Rose en Noir,* whose full and lusty heart hides a dark and brooding secret.

Zhivago, like Lara, would alternate his fragrances, but his motives would be different. While with his wife Tonya, he would wear CHANEL's sensuous and appealing *Allure Homme,* but when he was with Lara he would wear Malbrum's spiritual yet contrasted, *Shameless Seducer.*

Meanwhile, faithful and forgiving Tonya would wear only Cacharel's brilliantly warm and generous floral aldehydic fragrance, *Loulou.*

The urbane and impeccably dressed, Komarovsky, would change his fragrances depending upon the expediency of his current political or personal situation. When feeling secure and jovial, he would apply a heavy dose of Dior's suave citrus and rosemary *Eau Sauvage,* but when feeling threatened, he wouldn't hesitate to deploy Maison Le Galion's cruel and metallic cologne, *Whip.*

Even the radical, Pasha, would have changed his attitude towards perfume. Newly convinced of the revolutionary purity of Aether's *Muskethanol,* composed entirely of synthetic molecules, he would grant himself the luxury of being subdued by its beauty.

On another front, the 2002 film *Chicago* starring Catherine Zeta-Jones and Renée Zellweger is literally boiling over with some of the rowdiest 1920s prohibition-era Bad Girls you've ever seen – and they're all making war, not love! Unlike Zhivago's Lara, however, none of the Chicago Bad Girls have any regrets whatsoever for what they've done (except, of course, that they got caught). Meanwhile, clued in Bad Girls know that similarly to *Dr. Zhivago, Chicago* has a silent and invisible, yet incredibly rich back-story that's loaded with some of the greatest fragrances in perfume history, all playing out in loud and clashing olfactory cacophony.

Starting with the opening scene. Velma Kelly arrives late and in a frenzy at the stage entrance to the theatre, and we watch as she tosses a revolver into a trashcan. We hear her entrance music, and once she's in her dressing room, we observe her frantically washing blood off her hands while dressing for her number. A knock at the door. She's on in "two." Watch carefully now, and you'll understand. Velma is not washing off her fragrance. Her husband's fragrance. Former husband. The man she loved and has just murdered. In one defining moment, *Knize Ten* has become *her* fragrance. She wears it like an invisible trophy.

What we don't see in the film is what Velma smelled on her sister the day before while rehearsing their new "sister act." What she smelled was *betrayal* in the unmistakable scent of *Knize Ten*, considered by many to be one of the best leather compositions in history.

Neither do we see the first perfume *denouement,* when they, not Velma, had been surprised as she stormed into the dressing room and found them making love. Velma had to defend her turf, even if it meant destroying a part she had loved that was now fouled. Take no prisoners. Start with her cheating man. Next, her lying sister. No more innocence. Velma could take care of herself.

Finishing the job, Velma would have snatched up a bottle of *Knize Ten* so carelessly left on the vanity.

"This is mine, now. This is me. I have earned it!"
A fixed character, Velma never sways from her *Knize Ten.* Throughout the film we sense its classy, well-oiled precision in her every graceful and perfectly timed move. With nerves of steel, she's there on the first beat of her opening number, and carries off her act even as she sees the cops moving in on her through the audience.

Velma's nemesis, Roxie Hart, is a chameleon. Shifting and fickle, Roxie dreams of vaudeville glory. More precisely what she wants is Velma's life style, and she'll sleep her way to the top to get it. Her fragrance of choice is François Coty's 1905 "In Your Face" floral-oriental fragrance, *L'Origan* (the Golden One). That is, until the bottle is shattered, along with her glorious illusions, when she shoots her lover. In prison, on charges of murder and facing the prospects of an all male jury, Roxie is advised by her flamboyant flim-flam lawyer Billy Flynn (Richard Gere), to shift her tactic and adopts Houbigant's 1912 classy "Innocent Flower" fragrance *Quelques Fleurs* (a few flowers), a sumptuous multi-floral bouquet. Billy Flynn is, of course, wearing Creed's citrus and woody fragrance, *Bois de Cedrat.*

Meanwhile, Murderer's Row of the Cook County Jail for female prisoners reeks with a fragrance signature all its own. At one end of the cell block, the office of the gluttonous and lascivious prison matron, Mama Morton, (Queen Latifah) is redolent with the opulent "In Your Face" white floral notes of François Coty's *Jasmin de Corse* (Corsican Jasmine) which she constantly and obsessively applies from a bottle of heavy Baccarat crystal. Pulsing from the other end of the hall, is the feverish cell-block chant, "He Had it Coming." The rich and pungent, very human and musky notes of personal body odor all but block out the fragile yet hauntingly beautiful and persistent notes of "The Hunyak's" desperate solo assertion that she is "Not Guilty." But there can be no secrets on death row. Ultimately it is The Hunyak's fragrance, Jeanne Lanvin's *My Sin,* that gives her away.

For the fun and on a much lighter note, two other Bad Girls and their fragrances make cameo appearances at the prison. Kitty Baxter (Lucy Liu), the kick-ass Bad Girl millionaire heiress, bursts on the scene, fresh from killing her husband and his two mistresses, and briefly outshines Velma and Roxie. Kitty is, of course, wearing Guerlain's 1906 spicy and floral Oriental fragrance, *Après L'Ondée* (after the rain shower).

Meanwhile, the bright-faced sensationalist reporter, Mary Sunshine (Christine Baranski), is ever ready to top up the juiciest news of the day with personal interpretations and fantasies with Aqua di Parma's lively citrus fragrance, *Colonia.* For the record, this woman is as much of a Bad Girl murderess as all the rest. Her victim? Journalism.

◈ ◈ ◈

In *Chicago's* grand Finale, Velma and Roxie join forces having grudgingly recognize each other's excellent qualities as totally wily and shrewd Bad Girls. Now, one hell of a wildly successful deadly duo, they remain distinctly themselves – Velma exultant in her *Knize Ten,* while Roxie has finally become *Coty's L'Origan.*

If a contemporary director were rash enough to take on this warring gang of Chicago Bad Girls for a remake of the film, the fragrance credits would read something like this:

VELMA	J.F. Schwarzlose Berlin's *Treffpunkt 8 Uhr* beautifully contrasting masculine and feminine energies.
ROXIE	Michael Kors' *White,* sparkling and luxurious.
BILLY FLYNN	Lubin's *Upper 10,* wealth and clout.
MARY SUNSHINE	Clinique's *Happy,* bright and sunny.
MAMA MORTON	*Dior Addict,* sensual and insatiable.
KITTY BAXTER	Blackbird's *Pipe Bomb Intense,* metallic and fuming.

And singing the cell-block theme song, *He Had It Coming*
The Celebrity Fragrance Bad Girls Chorus

FEATURING:

SELENA GOMEZ	*Vivamore,* exotic and intoxicating.
JENNIFER LOPEZ	*Glow,* skin scent trail.
CHRISTINA AGUILERA	*Touch of Seduction,* irresistible sensuality.
BEYONCÉ	*Heat,* fiery and passionate.
MARIAH CAREY	*Dreams,* warm and delicious.
KATY PERRY	*Killer Queen,* powerful and rebellious.
BRITNEY SPEARS	*Fantasy,* provocative love potion.

Oh, la-la! Those poor Bad Boyfriends of the warring Chicago Bad Girls. They're in big trouble with all this headed their way.

I'm sure my Bad Girl readers agree that the motives of these newly recruited warring *Chicago* Bad Girls are as pure as those in the original production, and if there's anybody who disagrees, the only response is simply another round of the rousing chorus (louder this time), "HE HAD IT COMING!"

◈

◈ CHAPTER NINE ◈

Cool Under Fire

It is most important that we Bad Girls know how to keep cool. Even, and especially, when we've gotten into such a heap of trouble that it might really and truly seem to be the end of the world. This is the moment to keep cool. For our sanity, and more importantly, for our *persona*, the last thing we want anybody to know is that we're upset.

The French have an expression: *chercher quelqu'un* which literally means "to go out looking for somebody," but the expression is similar to "egging somebody on," or "trying to get a rise out of them by pushing their buttons." Well, Bad Girl, we need to recognize this as one of the most common and underhanded techniques our enemies might ever use against us. They correctly believe that getting us upset will throw us off our game. If we get upset, chances are we'll overheat, lose it, and then, well, at least for that agenda item, we're toast! I'm sure you've all got stories and maybe even a few scars to show from past overheating experiences....

That's why it's crucially important to be ready for this challenge, so you know just how to assure this jerk that you are not going to "lose it." In fact, you're going to baffle the entire world by being totally and unwaveringly cool.

By now, you've surely realized that your Bad Girl "friends in need" are perfumes, and you might have even guessed that the perfume heroines for keeping your cool are *colognes* – refreshing, centering, and essential. Perhaps, the most important thing about colognes is that they not only give the impression of freshness and coolness, they make you feel that way too. Very important.

Face it. If you're like me, over the course of a perfectly normal Bad Girl day, there might be several times when you feel as if you're going to bust a gusset over something. I know, I know. It's awful. Can be downright embarrassing. Or worse still – devastating. I've been there. But after years of experience I've come to accept this as one of the facts of a Bad Girl's life, and learned to prepare for this by always keeping one of my favorite colognes close at hand. This technique has saved my Bad Girl skin on more than one occasion.

Don't get me wrong. Colognes are not just for use in emergencies. It goes without saying that colognes are basic equipment for the best of hot summer days. There are also plenty of days throughout the year when I start out feeling great, and all I want is a dash of light perfume or cologne to maintain that wonderful feeling. But I'm also very careful to keep cologne handy, even in darkest winter. And you should too. Nobody wants to be caught *in extremis.* Overheating Bad Girl moments can strike 365.

And although I feel quite clever and smug on such occasions as I douse myself in my coolant of choice, I know I didn't just make up this cologne technique out of the blue. Not by a long shot. In fact, Bad Girls have been using perfumed coolants – cologne, eau de cologne, and eau de toilette (toilet water), etc., for centuries.

For your amusement and edification, and to help figure out which ones might be best for you, and in which circumstances (you'll need several), I've pulled together some of my favorite stories from the illustrious and ongoing history of Bad Girls Perfume in which colognes play a major role.

Just to make sure you know what we're talking about here, a cologne is a cocktail of fragrant materials (commonly made from the rinds of citrus fruits and aromatic plants) in a concentration of up to 4% in an alcohol and water base. Eau de Cologne is generally a 3-8% concentration, while Eau de Toilette is generally 5-15%. By comparison, Eau de Parfum, Pure Perfume, Perfume Extract (extrait de parfum) and Perfume (parfum) are 15-40% (average 25%).

There can be considerable variation and overlap in these concentrations and ingredients, and to make things more confusing, virtually all men's fragrances up until the late 1990s were referred to as colognes no matter what their concentration, primarily because other terms had feminine connotations.

Because of their rapid evaporation, colognes and eau de colognes give an immediate cooling and stimulating effect when applied to the skin, and by proxy, to the mood of the person using them. This is why, in addition to their cooling qualities, colognes are often associated with sensations of wellbeing, optimism, and even zestiness, which is derived from the French word *zeste*, meaning the rind of a citrus fruit.

For the sake of simplicity, unless specifically noted, I'll use the terms cologne, eau de cologne, cologne-type fragrance, eau de toilette, and toilet water interchangeably throughout this chapter whether referring to men's colognes, women's colognes, eau de toilette (toilet waters), light fragrances, or splashes.

Our Cologne story begins back in the 14th century, when a certain Bad Girl, Elizabeth of Poland, came into possession of a very interesting fragrance concoction. Referred to as *Eau de la Reine de Hongrie* (The Queen of Hungary's Cologne) for reasons you'll understand in a minute, this particular mixture was comprised primarily of rosemary oil and alcohol, and was created for our dear Elizabeth by a monk. He told her that it was an "elixir," a product with purported health benefits.

And so it was. Elizabeth of Poland claimed that in addition to being an important coolant, her *Eau de la Reine de Hongrie* was a mood and beauty enhancer, and remarkably beneficial to her health. She used it externally for "frictioning" (rubbing vigorously all over the body) and internally. Yep, you heard me right. She drank the stuff. Since the alcohol base of the elixir was similar to a wine or liqueur, internal and external usage of elixirs was common practice at the time. Cool, huh? Please do NOT try this at home with your colognes, though. Thanks to modern, supposedly protective (read, Bad Girl kill-joy) global norms and regulations, the alcohol component in all commercially sold cologne and perfume products have been "denatured," i.e., made to taste and digest horribly, cause vomiting, etc.. This, of course, is to prevent them from being used for "recreational" purposes. If you're like me you probably already know this, having at one time in your life, decided to give it a try. You may have even been inspired by Scarlet O'Hara's example when she used the old perfume gargling trick (unsuccessfully) to cover up her *drinking-alone Bourbon Breath,* one sunny morning when Rhett Butler happened to call on her unannounced. If you've done this, you now know better, and I don't need to worry about your trying it again. If you haven't done it, don't. Of course, I know you will, Bad

Girl, so please promise to only take a tiny sip. Trust me. And whatever you do, don't gargle.

Returning to the story of our Polish Bad Girl, Elizabeth, she claimed that her elixir healed her of a disfiguring and crippling disease, relieved her gout, rheumatism, and improved her libido. She couldn't have been lying about this part, because following her miraculous recovery from various impairments, the King of Hungary proposed to her. Some sources say she refused him; others say she accepted. Given the name of the formula, "The Queen of Hungary's Cologne," I'm betting she accepted, a fact which certainly would have intensified the other benefits of the formula and contributed to her long and happy life. For the record, Elizabeth is credited as being the first person to introduce perfume to Europe and the Western world. You go, Bad Girl!

Fast-forward to the 16th century court of France, where another infamous Bad Girl was set to spend a lifetime depending upon colognes and perfumes for coolants (and other less noble uses). In 1533, when fifteen-year Catherine de Medici left her native Florence, Italy, to become the bride of Henri Duke of Orleans, second son of Francis I of France, this girl was headed for *stress.* Luckily, for our young and future queen (mentioned earlier in *Chapter 5: The Huntress,* as the rival of Bad Girl Huntress, Diane de Poitiers), the Florentines at the time were arguably the most sophisticated perfume power on the Continent, and Catherine was armed to the gills. Not only did she arrive with her personal perfumer and an array of perfumed products, she possessed a secret weapon, *Acqua della Regina* (later known as *Acqua di Colonia*) created by the good friars of the Officina Profumo Farmaceutica Santa Maria Novella (AKA Santa Maria Novella, which is still thriving today) to honor the marriage of their Florentine princess.

It's true that in the short term, Catherine was unable to establish her power or win the heart of her husband, the King, from his mistress, Diane. If you remember correctly from *Chapter 5: The Huntress,* Diane was managing quite well, and continued to retain the upper hand in the affair by capitalizing on her superior skills as a huntress in conjunction with "Made in France" natural fragrance products, and her precious *Eau de la Reine de Hongrie.*

Though as volatile as the essences of her signature fragrance, Catherine was also quite cunning, knew the art of playing for the long game, and, as a Medici, was clever at assessing the stakes (a kingdom is worth more than a king, for example). While biding her time through years in Diane's shadow and lack of Kingly "attention," she certainly relied on frequent applications of her namesake *Acqua della Regina* to keep her cool and lift her spirits.

And then one fateful day, her husband, the king, died in a jousting accident, and the tables turned for our Bad Girl Catherine. Through schemes and machinations that would make a Renaissance courtier's hair stand on end, Catherine, now Queen Regent of France, managed to successively maintain two of her sons on the throne through years of bloody civil and religious wars. She also accomplished important things for the French perfume industry by introducing advanced Florentine fragrance techniques such as the art of perfuming gloves, thus helping to establish France and the city of Grasse as perfume capitals of the world. Perhaps, most importantly from a woman's point of view, our Bad Girl Catherine de Medici would have felt sweet revenge when she evicted Diane de Poitiers from the Chateau de Chenonceau, and reclaimed this most beautiful of chateaux for herself. "Now, it's *my* turn, my dear." In the profuse flow of blood, curses, poison, and intrigue that characterized Catherine de Medici's time of power, we can also imagine an ironically sweet and uplifting note, as if rising from gallons and gallons of *Acqua della Regina*. Clearly powerful stuff.

A century and a half later, yet another Florentine, Giovanni Paolo Feminis (1685-1766), was about to make a colossal impact on perfumery. Having immigrated to Cologne, Germany (then part of Prussia), the young Feminis developed a formula he called *Aqua Admirabilis Coloniae* (Admirable Eau de Cologne), composed of *esprit de vin* (distilled wine), citrus, floral, and aromatic notes, inspired by his native Italy, and a visit to Santa Maria Novella.

What became of Feminis' original formula is the subject of more legends than facts, and as there were no patent laws at the time, it didn't take long for numerous iterations of *Aqua Admirabilis Coloniae* to see the light of day. Meanwhile, at the end of the Napoleonic Wars (1803-1815), French soldiers returning from the occupied city of Cologne brought bottles of this *Aqua Admirabilis Coloniae* back with them to France. Tired of the heavier, musky fragrances of the time, and newly entranced with the art of bathing, French Bad Girls and Boys jumped on this new light fragrance and called it "Eau de Cologne." The name stuck. From this time forward, the term "Eau de Cologne" or simply "Cologne" came into common usage to designate perfumed products, generally containing a light concentration of citrus, herbal, and floral notes in an alcohol and water base.

In all of this, three contemporary colognes claim to be legitimate heirs of the original *Aqua Admirabilis Coloniae* formula.

In Cologne, Germany, *Farina 1709 Eau de Cologne Original* was created in 1709 by Feminis's nephew, Johann Maria Farina (upon the inspiration of Feminis' formula), and is still produced by the 8th generation of the Farina family. Also in Cologne, Mäurer & Wirtz's Eau de Cologne, *4711,* is based on a formula (purportedly that of Feminis) received as a gift to the family in 1792. Across the Rhine in France, Roget & Gallet's *Extra Vieille* traces its legitimacy to the original Feminis *Aqua Admirabilis Coloniae* via a younger Jean-Marie Farina, who arrived in Paris in 1806 in possession of a formula apparently inherited from his great-uncle.

More importantly, at least for our story, and perhaps *the* reason for its enormous success, Bad Girls and Boys across the world recognized colognes as the most "admirable" of cooling allies, and flocked to the counters of its purveyors. To add to the fun, while maintaining the name, Cologne, in reference to the citrus and aromatic ingredients of early formulas, individual perfumers began adding their own touches – a bit of amber here, a tad of Russian leather there, while at the same time playing with stronger and weaker concentrations of the fragrant products.

In Florence, the good friars of Santa Maria Novella, well established since the 13th century, and claiming no reference but their own illustrious history, continued to produce outstanding and sophisticated colognes, and in 1828 launched *Frangipane* with powdery and woody notes, *Garofano* of distinctive carnation and benzoin notes, and *Maresciallo,* an amazing chypre eau de cologne. Similar activities were taking place in monasteries throughout the peninsula, further highlighting Italy's central role in cologne history.

Never to be upstaged, and in a clear signal to the world

that France, too, is at the heart of cologne territory, Guerlain's founder Pierre-François Pascal Guerlain, created *Eau de Cologne Imperiale* in1853 for a powerful Bad Girl of note, Queen Eugenie, wife of Napoleon III. With its fresh citrus and rosemary notes, *Eau de Cologne Imperiale* was an immediate hit with Bad Girls and Boys throughout the courts of Europe.

At approximately the same time, colognes of another French perfume house, L.T. Piver, bearing grandly evocative names such as *L'Eau de Cologne des Princes,* achieved worldwide renown with such notable Bad Girls as French actress Sarah [Bernhardt] Bernard as well as with notoriously *bad* members of the Bonaparte family. Meanwhile, The House of Creed, founded in London in 1760 by James Henry Creed, and known for its classy men's colognes such as *Royal Scottish Lavender,* relocated to Paris in 1854 at the request of client Empress Eugenie of France, and created a namesake fragrance for her, *Jasmin Imperatrice Eugenie,* a fragrance still popular today.

Across the Channel, English colognes were speeding to the rescue of our Anglo-Saxon Bad Girl sisters, including none other than dear Miss Elizabeth Bennet of *Pride and Prejudice* fame. Oh yes, despite her outwardly demure appearances, the heroine of Jane Austen's 1813 landmark novel had no choice but to be a very, very Bad Girl (primarily "Undercover" though totally "Out There" when necessary), and therefore utterly dependent on the soothing powers of colognes. Whether dealing with the stress of property entailment, refusing a marriage proposal from a man she despised, or standing up to the wrath of one of the most powerful dowagers in her universe, Elizabeth would have relied on cooling and calming natural and commercial cologne-type fragrances as her constant allies while she managed to help one sister marry the love of her life, and, of course, find her own Mr. Darcy.

While Ms. Austen was not forthcoming about Elizabeth's fragrances in her novel, the BBC's 1995 TV mini-series of the same name offers glimpses of the Bennet sisters gathering lavender from the garden. Like all fine ladies of her time, Elizabeth would have kept sachets of lavender in her linen closets and drawers, and tucked under her pillow. It's not difficult to imagine the cool, assured, delicately biting, and oh so seductive fragrance of lavender rising from Elizabeth's ample bosom as she sings *Voi Che Sapete* to a visibly moved and nearly swooning Darcy. The disarmingly simple combination of colognes and soaps might well have been produced by a company established by the Cleaver family in 1770, which was to become the House of Yardley, famed for its array of English Lavender fragrances and toiletries.

Less than a half-century later, Elizabeth's compatriot, Florence Nightingale (1820-1910), was operating within the same system, but with other agenda items in mind, which she could never have accomplished without forging deeply into Bad Girl territory. A courageous social reformer, and credited as being the founder of modern nursing, Miss Nightingale spoke her mind and carried out her own plans, which among other things involved the scandal of traveling alone, as a single woman, to eastern Europe for hospital work during the Crimean War. Perhaps even more Bad, upon her return to England she set up the first training school for nurses, thus advancing all female well-being by opening the field of medicine to women through nursing. Oooooh! Really Bad, Florence, venturing into Male Territory like that. Oh yes, and she never married, although she had many admirers and was even engaged to one long-suffering suitor for nine years before breaking it off.

Through all of this we can be certain that our dear Miss Nightingale frequently called upon the soothing and cooling qualities of colognes. A letter she wrote in 1863 to the founder of Floris, thanking him for his "beautiful, sweet-smelling nosegays" (small bouquets popularly worn in Victorian England as fashion accessories) gives a hint as to the actual fragrances she might have worn. For her daily hospital rounds, she might have chosen *Floris Limes,* a classic citrusy and floral Eau de Toilette launched in 1832. And to help her endure the tedium of obligatory social engagements, peppered certainly with lectures about the importance of marriage, she might have chosen Floris's *White Rose,* a most deceptively innocent soft and green fragrance with just a hint of peppery "backtalk" from its carnation notes.

Across the Atlantic, the tale of a successful "Made in USA" cologne simply titled, *N°6,* is of curious significance in the unfolding story of the love affair between Bad Girls and colognes. With no claims to Farina's formula, *N°6* was first sold in 1752, miraculously survived the American Revolution, and remains popular today. Herein lies an excellent Bad Girls Perfume story, but you'll have to wait till the end of it to understand why.

In 1752 Dr. William Hunter, a Scottish immigrant pharmacist, founded a company he would call Caswell-Massey, and created a cologne called *N°6,* which became a favorite of George Washington, perhaps because its spicy blend of bergamot, florals, and aromatics seemed to embody the American spirit. Legend has it that George Washington even offered a case of *N°6* to Lafayette in thanks for helping the Americans win their independence. The irony of the story is that at the conclusion of the war, poor old Dr. Hunter found himself on the wrong side of things, was arrested for his Tory (pro-British) leanings, and run out of town on a rail. It was his wife, who managed to save the company through God knows what machinations. I've never read anything about the worthy Mrs. Hunter, but she must have been one hell of a Bad Girl to have skillfully constructed the kind of "Two Faces of Eve" persona it would have taken to navigate the razor's edge between the opposing forces of her husband's (and maybe her own) Tory beliefs, and the feverish Independent spirit of her clients, the newly minted citizens of the United States of America.

Not to forget another American Bad Girl cologne cousin, *Florida Water* (sometimes known as *Kanuga Water*), though of humbler origins, was in common usage and production at the same time. With a similar citrus base, *Florida Water's* name refers to the fabled Fountain of Youth, said to be located in Florida. In addition to its refreshing qualities, and containing the native American sweet orange rather than the neroli (bitter orange) of European colognes, *Florida Water* is purported to own magical healing and rejuvenating properties, and has been associated with voodoo and other magical and ritualistic ceremonies since the get-go. We can be sure that Marie Laveau (1794-1881), the infamous Creole Bad Girl Voodoo Queen and brothel matron, would have included some iteration of *Florida Water* (along with her magical snake "Zombie") in the legendary rites and divinations she performed during the course of her colorful career. A commercial form of *Florida Water* by the brand Murray & Lanman is available today in shops in North America and South America, along with other accouterments for similar practices.

Meanwhile, back on the Old Continent the warm and sunny life force of cologne continued to blossom in what many consider its native Italian soil. In 1853, Aqua di Genova presented its first colognes including, *Aqua di Genova Genes.* Less than twenty years later, the year 1871 saw the first edition of what was to become a well-beloved classic, *Acqua di Biella No.1* by the brand, Acqua di Biella.

In England, perhaps in compensation for a lesser degree of sunshine, William Penhaligon established his brand Penhaligon's in 1870, and in 1872 launched *Hammam Bouquet,* inspired by the sulfurous steam and exotic spices associated with Turkish baths, so popular among British upper classes of the time.

And that's just the beginning of things, girlfriends. Indeed, the popularity of colognes and toilette waters has done nothing but gather steam throughout the twentieth and twenty-first centuries, in spite of (or perhaps because of) the fact that until recently, many colognes were marketed as men's fragrances. As we saw in Chapter 4: ~~*Beg, Borrow, or*~~ Steal, any attempt to demarcate products as somehow belonging in "Men's" territory, only seems to incite Bad Girls to covet and steal them for their own iniquitous purposes. All the better, it appears, because it's SO much fun to steal from the "Gods," whether sneaking a splash of Papa's or Grand-Papa's *sent-bon* as the French call it, or waking up with it second-hand following a night of *Close [masculine] Encounters of [more than] the Third Kind.*

By the first decade of the 20th century, in addition to its positive vivacity, cologne had more than proven its adventurous globe-trotting spirit. Turns out a form of *Florida Water* even found its way to China in 1908 as *Two Girls,* thus offering indisputable proof that the powers of cologne had now reached global proportions. Just imagine: Two American *Florida Water* girls hanging out in Turn-of-the-Century China. The very idea shouts Bad Girls Perfume.

Meanwhile, the versatility and universal appeal of lavender continued to shine through in Penhaligon's 1910 lavender and clover *English Fern* with its clean and brisk British tone, while Aqua di Parma's 1916 lavender and citrusy *Colonia Acqua di Parma,* cast a Mediterranean light on the age old formula. What's more, the success of *Colonia Acqua di Parma,* especially among such Bad Girls (and Boys) as Ava Gardner, Audrey Hepburn, Cary Grant, and David Niven was living proof that not even a world war could interfere with the indomitable spirit of cologne.

Even during the 1920s when you might think that the newly liberated flappers had little need or desire to cool down from the un-corseted freedom they enjoyed, overheating moments were bound to erupt. Victor Margueritte's 1922 seminal novel, *La Garçonne* (The Flapper) describes in great (and scandalous) detail the life of one such Parisian flapper, Monique Lerbier, and her need to seriously cool down on more than one occasion over the course of her "career." There can be no doubt, for example, that following the devastating discovery that her fiancé was two-timing her, it would have taken more than a few hundred milliliters of cologne to quench the fire of her fury. Before leaping for cover, I might venture to suggest this might have been a hasty mix of several bottles snatched from her dresser, doused on her body, and then violently dashed to the floor. Among the chards her maid would have swept up in the aftermath, only a few names would have been decipherable, *Eau de Cologne Ambrée* by Jn. Giraud Fils (Grasse-Paris) perhaps, or *Oeillet* by Jardins de France. Others would have been splintered beyond recognition. For *La Petite histoire,* the shock wave this novel sent through proper French society was so great that it cost the author his prestigious place in the French Legion of Honor. How dare he so candidly suggest that a proper young woman, the very *fleur* of the French *haute bourgeoisie,* might be such a Bad Girl! Poor man, definitely a stalwart champion of our cause, he clearly knew a thing or two. Count this one up as a casualty of unfortunate "collateral damage" in the war of Bad Girls/Bad Boys against the World.

Colognes of the 1930s provided essential coolants and stress relievers for Bad Girls and Bad Boys during the Depression years. Caron's minimalistic *Pour Un Homme,* while offering a noble illustration of abundance in simplicity, was a reminder that class is the only essential; Dunhill's woody and leathery *Dunhill for Men* recalled the significance of rare and stolen moments shared between harried colleagues or lovers in the intimacy of a private smoke; Dana's sensual and musky *Canoe* seems to have been made for letting off the singular steam of a high school romance, in the back seat of Papa's Oldsmobile; and the Shulton Company's bright and oh so reassuring *Old Spice* (1938) was for everybody's Daddy's girl, trusting and optimistic against all odds.

Unbeknownst to many, the histories of two colognes created in the 1940s were intertwined with the lives and stories of several Bad Girls and Boys of the time. Indeed, a particular Bad Girl, Hollywood movie queen Ava Gardner, was associated with the green and mossy *Agua Lavanda,* launched in 1940 by the Spaniard Antonio Puig, as well as the fresh and citrusy *Green Water,* launched in 1947 by French Fashion designer Jacques Fath. As it turns out, *Agua Lavanda,* happened to be crooner Frank Sinatra's favorite splash at the time, and may well have been the spark that ignited a major sex scandal surrounding the love affair between Ava and Frank. It seems that Ava couldn't get enough of Sinatra, nor of his *Agua Lavanda.*

Meanwhile, Bad Girl Ava, not one to let grass grow under her feet, was apparently pouring it on elsewhere, as well. Notably, as a client of Jacques Fath, she was surely enjoying a splash or two of Fath's *Green Water* along with some of Fath's other Hollywood Bad Girl clients, Greta Garbo and Rita Hayworth. Whether any of Ava's *Green Water* ever rubbed off on loverboy Frank, is a matter of supposition. Suffice to say that the hot and tumultuous Gardner/ Sinatra love affair was the stuff of gossip columns for years to come.

Pour la petite histoire, Antonio Puig's perfume dynasty continues to thrive today and is responsible for the licensing of many outstanding Bad Girls cologne and fragrance brands, notably, Pacco Rabanne, Carolina Herrera, Comme des Garçons, Prada, Penhaligon's, and L'Artisan Parfumeur.

Meanwhile, Jacques Fath, considered to be one of the dominant forces in post-World War II *haute couture* (along with Christian Dior and Pierre Balmain), was also known to be quite charming and had a particular appeal for Bad Girls. Sadly, Fath died prematurely at the peak of his career, or God knows what other stories he might have contributed to history of Bad Girls Perfume. RIP.

The 1950s continued in the tradition of spicy and citrusy men's fragrances with classics such as *Eau d'Hermès,* Dior's *Eau Fraîche,* and *Monsieur de Givenchy,* all well-loved by Bad Girls for first and second-hand wearing. Meanwhile, three great perfume houses came to the rescue of Bad Girl Huntresses sweating it out in jungles and savannas across the world by bringing the dry, green-brown woody note of vetiver (a beach grass) to the cologne formula, each with their (almost) identically named fragrances, Carven's *Vetiver,* Guerlain's *Vetiver* (1961), and Givenchy's *Eau de Vetyver.* On another front, word went out on the Bad Girls Perfume Vine that *CHANEL Pour Monsieur,* CHANEL's first fragrance for men, was signaling a suspicious shift in what men were up to. Apparently no longer content to simply smell good and fresh, it seemed these guys were actually stealing some of our own Bad Girls Perfume techniques, and sending more complex and subtle messages. Oooooh, how dare they. Though certainly citrusy and spicy, *CHANEL Pour Monsieur,* also contained a hint of sultry chypre darkness, and was sometimes even referred to as an "intelligent" fragrance. Did these guys know more about Bad Girls than they were letting on? Considering the men Coco Chanel hung out with – seasoned Bad Boys such as Picasso, Stravinsky, and Cocteau – chances are likely they did. High Alert in the Bad Girls camp.

At the end of the decade, Bad Girls determined to "Make War, Not Love" certainly gnashed their teeth at Bad Boy Charles Revson's new Revlon cologne *That Man,* deliberately named to *chercher* his brand rival, Elizabeth Arden. Apparently, Ms. Arden hated Mr. Revson's guts so much that she couldn't even be brought to speak his name, and only referred to him (in public, at least) as "That Man." Though Revson could surely imagine what she called him in private, social niceties prevented him from naming his fragrance "That Bastard." *Quand meme!* Apparently, only the tip of the iceberg of what was surely a pitched battle among Bad Girls and Boys in the Fragrance Zone.

In the frenzied jungle of the 1960s Sexual Revolution, Dior essentially defined the conditions on the ground with *Eau*

Sauvage, while Lubin acknowledged the colossal sea change at hand with *Eau Neuve* (new water). Meanwhile, seizing an unprecedented opportunity, Santa Maria Novella nailed the mood of the era for Bad Girls *and* Boys by marketing its new *Melograno* fragrance with its pomegranate tartness as "unisex." At approximately the same time, Diptyque opened the doors of its shop on the Boulevard Saint-Germain in Paris, and launched its first eau de toilette, *L'Eau,* which like all its fragrances was "unisex," as well. Reflecting another trend of the 60s, the importance of equality among social and economic classes, the budget-priced French cologne brand, Bien-Être, might well have had as its motto, "Not a Bad Girl left behind!" when it launched its landmark *Eau de Cologne Naturelle.* Uncomplicated, reasonably priced, and accessible to all in supermarkets and pharmacies, this *sent-bon* remains dear to the hearts of French Bad Girls and Bad Boys across all generations and classes.

Meanwhile, in the 1970s two new companies caught the mood of nature-loving Bad Girls, and their bathing and toilet needs from colognes to soaps to shampoos. In France, L'Occitane En Provence, and in the UK, The Body Shop, (now part of L'Oréal,) specialized in naturally-scented soaps and lotions. Both were also early proponents of products of Fair Trade origin inspired by nature.

Among the numerous fashion brands launching colognes or toilette waters in the 70s, Yves Saint Laurent certainly thrilled many a Bad Girl AND Bad Boy by challenging social taboos and posing naked in the ads for his *Pour Homme.* Closing out the decade, Hermès called on master Bad Girl perfumer, Françoise Caron to create *Eau de Cologne Hermès,* (later baptised *Eau d'Orange Verte*), reflecting the shifts and contrasts of the times through the brightness and effervescence of citrus notes, and the dark moodiness of oak moss and patchouli chypres notes.

Among the outstanding colognes and light fragrances created in the 1980s, Diptyque's *L'Ombre Dans L'Eau* (shadow in the water) was a cunning nod to Bad Girl Witches and the dark side, with its hauntingly beautiful harmony of black currant leaf and Bulgarian rose. Giorgio Armani's *Armani Eau Pour Homme* set the gold standard for Bad Girl Huntresses in search of floral, woody colognes they might run to ground on their boyfriends' bodies, or simply bag for themselves. And the fresh, sharp sea notes of *Cool Water* by Davidoff, so popular with guys of the 15-25 year-old set, will forever echo in the treacherous songs of the Bad Girl Mermaids who love them, or pretend to.

Meanwhile, the Spa craze that took over Bad Girls territory in the 1980s and 90s inspired an entirely new category of colognes, "Treatment Fragrances," with the 1987 launch of Clarins' *Eau Dynamisante,* a spicy and refreshing chypre. In the tradition of "elixers" (mentioned earlier in this chapter, regarding *L'Eau de la Reine de Hongrie*) Clarins "Treatment Fragrances" claim therapeutic benefits, such as skin softening and toning, along with cooling and aromatic properties. In a similar vein, the American brand, Bath & Body Works with a goal of helping customers improve their emotional and physical wellbeing through simple and pleasurable rituals of daily self-care, was a clear call to Bad Girls in need of SPA-type pampering. Meanwhile, Elizabeth Arden, catering to the same Bad Girl population's search for coolants of the body, mind, and soul, even threw in a gourmand treat when she brought out *Green Tea,* an invigorating and aromatic "Scent Spray."

In 1994, Jo Malone opened her first boutique, and suggested that clients layer her simple and light fragrances and colognes.

In the last decade of the century, the venerable old cologne formula proved its capacity for maintaining sex-appeal in classic iterations, as well as in new formulations reflecting evolving times. Lorenzo Villoresi's 1996 *Acqua di Colonia* was successful as a deliberate throw-back to the classic citrus and rosemary of the *Eau de la Reine de Hongrie* formula. At the same time Calvin Klein's 1994 uni-sex *ck One,* in a clear forward look to the new frontiers of the 21st century, poured even more musk notes – both erotic and clean – into the traditional cologne formula, and literally cornered the youth market of Bad Girls and their Bad Boy friends.

Just to prove that cool was getting hotter and hotter even beyond the world of cologne, Donna Karan came out with an EdP, *DKNY Women* whose delivery was so cool, it was downright cold – imitating the icy punch of a vodka cocktail, another Bad Girl coolant of choice. And for purists, *L'Eau par Kenzo For Women* offered the sensation of pure water, cooled with just a touch of frosted mint.

In the last year of the century, building on what was now more than a hundred years of experience in satisfying Bad Girls' need for coolants, Guerlain caught on to yet another crying Bad Girls Perfume need: Simplicity. Indeed, the Guerlain team had correctly read a chorus of Bad Girls Perfume lips chanting, "**K**eep **I**t **S**imple, **S**tupid!" when it created the *Aqua Allegoria* eau de toilette line with its deliberately simple formulas. Great news for over-heated and overworked Bad Girls. Not surprisingly, the wildly successful Guerlain "Kiss Kiss" lipstick collection was only a few years away.

In the opening years of the 21st century, the rising tide of colognes in Bad Girls territory has reached record levels, and as of this "Beach Watch" shows no sign of abating. As colognes, toilette waters, or mere splashes, the waves continue to pour in – alone, in pairs, or sometimes, like Comme des Garçons's 2002 *Cologne Séries 4,* (gulp!) in series.

Bad Girls now have the widest choice of cooling colognes ever. No risk of global warming in this fragrant ecosystem. In fact, the biggest danger for Bad Girls these days is not that they might overheat, but rather that they might drown! Undaunted, even as the waves have taken on the proportions of tsunamis, Bad Girls have simply brought out their surfboards.

The waves may be bigger, but the water is decidedly lighter. The touch of CHANEL's *Cristalle Eau Verte,* for example, is even softer than CHANEL's *Cristalle.* The heavy clank of coins in Paco Rabanne's EdP, *1 Million,* has become an engaging tinkle in *1 Million Cologne.* And you've got to know something big is going on when even the ideal man lightens up. Well, he has. Guerlain's 2015 *L'Homme Ideal Cologne* has a noticeably lighter style than *L'Homme Ideal EdP* from only a year before.

Bigger yes. Lighter yes. Any chance of something even more varied and wild? Yes. Whatever you want, Bad Girls, we've got it. There are even more sensual musks in Thierrry Mugler's *Cologne.* There's cassis, musk, and white amber in Cartier's *L'Eau de Cartier.* There's something bitter and metallic in Frédéric Malle's *Cologne Bigarde.* There are even marine notes in Ralph Lauren's *Blue.*

What's more, these lighter, wilder colognes are no longer content to simply offer us a refreshing morning kiss. Ever eager to please, they now want to be with us twenty-four hours a day. Maison Francis Kurkdjian has gone so far as to offer us colognes for morning and evening with *Cologne pour la Matin* and *Cologne pour le Soir,* while Le Galion gives us *Cologne* and *Cologne Nocturne.*

No doubt about it, Bad Girl, these cologne dudes are after our bods. Indeed, in their territorial urges, some even seem ready to go to war with their kinsmen, perfumes. The arrival of Serge Lutens' aldehydic and musky *L'Eau* in 2009, for example, is sometimes touted as an "anti-perfume." Could there be some kind of battle for our bodies going on?

Reminds me of Guinevere, that Bad Girl of all Bad Girls, who in the story of Camelot, single-handedly busted up King Arthur's Knights of the Round Table. Those who know the story will surely remember that, among other things, the worthy Queen Guinevere fantasized about the possibility that "kith might kill their kin" for her.

Mais, non! No no no no, et non. Although the idea might be titillating as a fantasy, this is not at all what Guinevere really wanted. She loved and needed both men, Arthur and Lancelot, passionately and totally – for different reasons. Likewise, Bad Girls love and need many perfumes and colognes for myriad reasons, some of which they're only just discovering. The last thing Bad Girls want is for their fragrance lovers to kill each other off. *Au contraire.* They want to have them all, very much alive, and all at once, *s'il vous plait!*

Impossible? Not at all. Any Bad Girl worth her salt knows that if she wants a miracle, she need only ask for the unattainable. Indeed, in 2009, as if in answer to a collective Bad Girls Perfume prayer, the Franco-American brand, Atelier Cologne, burst on the scene like an Action Hero offering fragrances with the freshness of cologne and the staying power of perfume. Atelier Cologne's original fragrance, *Orange Sanguine,* offers clear references to the citrus and sunny heart of colognes, while fragrances in subsequent Atelier Cologne collections continue to strike a perfume/cologne balance in the *Cologne Absolue* formula, defined by the brand as, "…a neo-classic perfume which blends the elegance of citruses with the most precious raw materials in perfumery."

To top things off, Atelier Cologne accompanies its "hybrid" fragrances with enticing, life-imitating-art, back-stories (on and off the record). Each fragrance has a highly developed, romantic, and intriguing personality, whose story, complete with images, reads like a pulp fiction novelette. Current favorites of this Bad Girl, are the infamous duo, *Rose Anonyme,* a seductive international jewel thief, and *Vétiver Fatal,* the secret agent who loves her. Oooh! Absolute Bad Girl Fantasy land from top to bottom.

Following Atelier Cologne's challenge to the rigid barriers separating perfumes and colognes, Bad Girls can now enjoy unprecedented perfume and cologne freedom. While maintaining long and short-term relationships with their perfume lovers, they can dally with as many cologne lovers as they desire, or, as another option, find one or several that can go both ways.

Currently, with colognes coming on so strong, many of my Bad Girl friends are approaching this succession of men, er, I mean colognes, the same way they do a "one-night stand." Nothing serious please, just give me an occasion to indulge my senses with no thought for tomorrow. Where previously she might have blamed her coolant needs on the heat, the moment, the summer, or whatever the hell she felt like, today's Bad Girl doesn't even look for an excuse beyond the whims of her delightfully fickle nature. She obsesses. She exults. She moves on. There have been others. There will be more. No commitment. No (undesirable) consequences. Ah, is this not a perfect Bad Girls perfume life?

Seen in this light, the cologne brand Third Man, offers an example of how this new "dating game" works. Launched in 2011, Third Man first brought us *Eau Moderne,* then *Eau Monumentale,* then *Eau Profounde,* and now there's a 4th Third Man, and he's *Eau Nomade.* Gotta love it.

Meanwhile, many Bad Girls are wondering what to make of Frédéric Malle's 2015 *Cologne Indélébile* (Indelible/ Permanent Cologne). Are we to take this apparent oxymoron as a challenge? Are colognes and Bad Girls being asked to stick around? To be faithful? Or, like Atelier Cologne, could *Cologne Indélébile* simply be suggesting a redefinition of terms? If "cologne" can be redefined, can "fidelity" be redefined as well? Is a jolt of total, obsessive, absolutely focused fidelity for an hour or a day as valid or real as a lifetime's worth? Bad Girls are cogitating.

Meanwhile, don't go away. The story's not over yet. Always in need of coolants, Bad Girls clearly love the undeniable quality, sincerity, and *size* of current cologne offerings. And although they might no longer believe in the idea of one Mr. Right made in Perfume Heaven, a lot of them are finding what they're looking for with several Mr. Rights made in Cologne.

◈

◈ CHAPTER TEN ◈

The End of the World

Whatever their longevity on our bodies, and whether we choose, as with our lovers, to believe or not believe their lies about not trying to trick or trap us, colognes *and* perfumes have clearly wooed and won their rightful places in Bad Girls' hearts.

Whatever their intentions or strengths, all fragrances are our vital partners in this world thanks to their irreplaceable powers to conjure and highlight memories, dreams, and desire, and to transform, heat up, or cool down, our most cherished Bad Girls personas and fantasies.

How we choose to deploy them brings us to the very crux of the Bad Girls Perfume matter. Humor, that other great master of transformation, stress management, and solution finding, is also what makes Bad Girls invincible and irresistible. Whether open, light, and sparkling, or hidden, dark, and acerbic, humor is the ultimate Bad Girls trick and perfume technique. Linked to our volatile imagination and appreciation of the absurd, Bad Girls humor allows us to recognize the supposed flaws of life as nothing less than essential. To fight, or try to change them is to die. To accept and embrace them is to live. Some twist or quirk, some existential imbalance or imperfection that creates enigma is central to humor and to the perfumes we choose.

One of my favorite perfumes is Etat Libre d'Orange's *La Fin Du Monde* (The End of The World), because its quirky popcorn note is a perfect reminder of the central element of humor in the best of Bad Girls perfumes.

As Bad Girls, we *will* have the last laugh even when faced with the biggest bugaboo of them all, "The End of the World." Our mother, Eve, set us on course in Chapter One with a gutsy opening number, the least we can do is offer her an equally spirited grand finale.

How do we do this? Through Bad Girls Perfume fantasies, of course. Using perfume's transformative powers we simply imagine The End of the World as nothing more disturbing than one of our favorite Armageddon flicks, which we *enjoy* while hanging out with our buddies at the movies. Hey, it's The End of the World! Cool, huh? We're relaxed, sitting back, feet up on the seats in front of us, (maybe even kicking a few heads – oh, sorry!) and eating a bag of popcorn.

Worst case scenario? Turns out it's not The End of the World. Thanks to the power of perfume, if and when that moment ever arrives, we Bad Girls will be above and beyond it all, dousing ourselves in our favorite fragrances, and enjoying a really good (last) laugh.

And that's all there is to it, Bad Girl. From the Garden of Eden to the End of the World, we and our *Bad Girls Perfume* have definitely covered the *Territory.* After this, I think you'd agree: We can handle anything.

On this uplifting note, dear Bad Girl friend, I'll bid you farewell, and take my exit in a spritz of my favorite fragrance. It's your turn to write the next chapter in the fabulous history of *Bad Girls Perfume*, which as you undoubtedly know by now, is your own.

End

◈

◈ EPILOGUE ◈

After the End of the World

Hey, I knew you'd turn the page. Who but an absolute ace Bad Girl would know there's more to *Bad Girls Perfume* after The End of the World. Of course, there is.

Check out the scene at www.badgirlsperfume.com and add your stories to the surreal next chapter(s). You'll find yourself in good company.

◈

◈ BAD GIRLS PERFUME BAR ◈

Perfumes Referenced in *Bad Girls Perfume*

CHAPTER 1
BAD GIRLS NEED PERFUME

CHANEL *CHANEL N°5* 1921
Perfumer Ernest Beaux

Guerlain *Shalimar* 1925
Perfumer Jacques Guerlain

Dana *Tabu* 1932
Perfumer Jean Carles

Revlon *Jean Naté* 1935
Perfumer Ernest Shiftan

Guerlain *Jicky* 1889
Perfumer Aimé Guerlain

CHAPTER 2
THE TWO FACES OF EVE

Creed *Fantasia de Fleurs* 1862
Perfumer Henry Creed
Third Generation

Guerlain *Eau de Cologne Impériale* 1860
Perfumer Pierre-François-Pascal
Guerlain

Yardley *Rose* or *Violet*

Floris *White Rose* 1800

Molinard *Rose* 1860

Lubin *Rose Liberty*

Yves Saint Laurent *Paris* 1983
Perfumer Sophia Grojsman

Yves Rocher *Rose Fraiche* 2012
Perfumer Shyamala Maisondieu

A Lab on *Fire Rose Rebelle Respawn* 2013
Sophia Grojsman

Dear Rose *I Love My Man* 2014
Perfumer Fabrice Pellegrin

Xerjoff *Damarose* 2010
Perfumer Jacques Flori

The Different Company
I Miss Violet 2015
Perfumer Bertrand Duchaufour

Kenzo *Flower by Kenzo* 2000
Perfumer Alberto Morillas

L'Artisan Parfumeur kid gloves
scented with Mûre et Musc Extrême
(blackberries and musk) 1978
Perfumer Jean Laporte

CHAPTER 2 *(continued)*
THE TWO FACES OF EVE

Lubin *Gin Fizz* 1955
Perfumer Henri Giboulet and actualized 2009 Thomas Fontaine

Creed *Fleurissimo* 1956
Perfumer James Henry Creed Fifth Generation

Estée Lauder *Beautiful* 1985

Ralph Lauren *Romance* 1998
Perfumer Harry Fremont

Aedes de Venustas
Oeillet Bengale 2014
Perfumer Rodrigo Flores-Roux

Robert Piguet *Fracas* 1948
Perfumer Germaine Cellier

Coty *Truth or Dare* 2012
Perfumer Stephen Nilsen

Jeroboam *Hauto* 2015
Perfumer Vanina Muracciole

Nasomatto *Narcotic V/Narcotic Venus* 2007
Perfumer Alessandro Gualtieri

Editions de Parfums Frédéric Malle
Carnal Flower 2005
Perfumer Dominique Ropion

Histoires de Parfums
Tubereuse 2 Virginale 2010
Perfumers Sylvie Jourdet and Gérald Ghislain

Maria Christofilis *Fleur* 09 2012
Perfumer Rodrigo Flores-Roux

Dior *Diorissimo* 1956
Perfumer Edmond Roudnitska

Frédéric Malle *1er Mai* 2010
Perfumer Dominique Ropion

Etat Libre d'Orange *Don't Get Me Wrong Baby, I Don't Swallow* 2007
Perfumer Antoine Maisondieu

Narciso Rodriguez
Narciso Rodriguez for Her 2003
Perfumers Christine Nagel and Francis Kurkdjian

Lisa Hoffman Beauty
Tunisian Neroli 2007
Perfumer Ellen Molner

Le Labo *Lys 41* 2013
Perfumer Daphne Bugey

Jovoy *Gardez-Moi* Gardenia 2013
Perfumer Bertrand Duchaufour

Tom Ford *Velvet Gardenia* 2007
Perfumer Dave Apel

Julian Bedel
Agua Magnoliana 2010
Perfumer Julian Bedel

Grandiflora *Magnolia Grandiflora Michel* 2014
Perfumer Michel Roudnitska

Caron *Narcisse Noire* 1911
Perfumer Ernest Daltroff

Thierry Blondeau
Narcisse Émoi 2015
Perfumer Thierry Blondeau

Serge Lutens *À La Nuit* 2000
Christopher Sheldrake

Etat Libre d'Orange
Jasmin et Cigarette 2006
Perfumer Antoine Maisondieu

Annick Goutal *Passion* 1983
Perfumer Annick Goutal

By Kilian *Voulez-Vous Coucher Avec Moi* 2012 Alberto Morillas

Francis Kurkdjian
Absolue Pour Le Soir 2010
Perfumer Francis Kurkdjian

Jean Patou *JOY* 1930
Perfumer Henri Alméras

Prudence Paris *Nuits Blanches* 2014

Neela Vermeire Creations
Pichola 2015
Perfumer Bertrand Duchaufour

April Aromatics *Lindenblossom*
(Unter den Linden)
Perfumer Tanja Bochnig

Lubin *Upper Ten For Her* 2016
Perfumer Delphine Thierry

Givenchy *Organza* 1996
Perfumer Sophie Labbé

CHANEL *CHANEL N°5* 1921
Perfumer Ernest Beaux

Lanvin *Arpège* 1927
Perfumer Andre Fraysse

Dolce & Gabanna *D&G* 1992

Jean-Louis Scherrer *Scherrer 2* 1986
Perfumer Alberto Morillas

Andy Tauer *Noontide Petals* 2013
Perfumer Andy Tauer

Rochas *Madame Rochas* 1960 Guy Robert

Paco Rabanne *Calandre 1969*
Perfumer Michel Hy

Yves Saint Laurent
Rive Gauche 1971
Perfumer Michel Hy

Le Galion *Sortilège* 1936
Perfumer Paul Vacher; 2014
Perfumer Marie Duchene

Lancôme *Magie Noire* 1978
Perfumer Gerard Goupy

Cacharel *Loulou* 1987
Perfumer Jean Guichard

Coty *Emeraude* 1921
Perfumer François Coty

Guerlain *Shalimar* 1925
Perfumer Jacques Guerlain

Estee Lauder *Youth Dew* 1953
Perfumer Josephine Catapano

Yves Saint Laurent's *Opium* 1977
Perfumers Jean Amic and
Jean-Louis Sieuzac

Beverly Hills
Giorgio Beverly Hills 1981
Perfumers M.L. Quince,
Francis Camail, and Harry Cuttle

Dior *Poison* 1985
Perfumer Edouard Flechier

Calvin Klein *Obsession* 1985
Perfumer Jean Guichard

Beyoncé *Heat* 2010
Perfumers Claude Dir and
Olivier Gillotin

Serge Lutens *Féminité du Bois*
Perfumers Christopher Sheldrake
and Pierre Bourdon

Tom Ford *Black Orchid* 2006

Francis Kurkdjian
Lumière Noire 2009
Perfumer Francis Kurkdjian

Aqua di Parma 'Oud' shampoo

Tom Ford 'Oud Wood Bar' soap

Serge Lutens *Ambre Sultan* 2000
Perfumer Christopher Sheldrake

Annick Goutal *1001 Ouds* 2015
Perfumer Camille Goutal

Byredo *Seven Veils* 2011
Perfumer Jerome Epinette

Beverly Hills
Giorgio Beverly Hills 1981
Perfumers M.L. Quince, Francis Camail, and Harry Cuttle

Giulietta Capuleti *Far from the Balcony* 2014

CHAPTER 3
THE SEDUCTRESS

Coty *Chypre* 1917
Perfumer François Coty

Guerlain *Mitsouko* 1919
Perfumer Jacques Guerlain

Dior *Diorama* 1949
Perfumer Edmond Roudnitska

Weil *Zibeline* 1928
Perfumer Claude Fraysse

Carven *Ma Griffe* 1946
Perfumer Jean Carles

Hermès *Calèche* 1961 Guy Robert

Ungaro *Diva* 1983
Perfumer Jacques Polge

Schiaparelli *Shocking* 1937
Perfumer Jean Carles

Robert Piguet *Bandit* 1944
Perfumer Germaine Cellier

CHANEL *CHANEL N°19* 1970
Perfumer Henri Robert

CHANEL Les Exclusifs
31 rue Cambon 2007
Perfumer Jacques Polge

Serge Lutens *Rose de Nuit* 1993
Perfumer Gilles Romey

Sisley *Soir de Lune* 2006
Perfumer Dominique Ropion

Aqua di Parma
Iris Nobile EDP 2006
Perfumers Françoise Caron and Francis Kurkdjian

James Heeley *Hippie Rose* 2011

MDCI *Chypre Palatin* 2012
Perfumer Bertrand Duchaufour

Corday *Toujours Moi*
(Forever Me) 1924

Salvatore Ferragamo
Golden Acacia 2014

Guerlain *L'Heure Bleue* 1912
Perfumer Jacques Guerlain

Prada *Infusion de Fleur d'Oranger* 2009
Perfumer Daniela (Roche) Andrier

Vero Profumo *Rubj* 2007
Perfumer Vero Kern

Lanvin *Arpège* 1927
Perfumer Andre Fraysse

Dolce&Gabbana *D&G* 1992
Perfumer IFF

Jean-Louis Scherrer
Scherrer 2 1986
Perfumer Alberto Morillas

Tauer Perfumes
Noontide Petals 2013
Perfumer Andy Tauer

Houbigant *Quelques Fleurs L'Original* 1913
Perfumer Robert Bienaime

CHANEL *Misia* 2015
Perfumer Olivier Polge

CHANEL *CHANEL N°5* 1921
Ernest Beaux

Eight&Bob *Eight & Bob* 1937
Albert Fouquet

Guerlain *Mitsouko* 1919
Perfumer Jacques Guerlain

Pierre Balmain *Vent Vert* 1947
Germaine Cellier/Calice Becker

Clinique *Aromatics Elixir* 1971
Perfumer Bernard Chant

The Different Company
Sublime Balkiss 2008
Perfumer Celine Ellena

Ulrich Lang New York
Aperture 2014

Nomenclature *Adr-ett* 2015
Perfumer Frank Voelkl

Paloma Picasso
Paloma Picasso 1984
Perfumer Francis Bocris

Molinard *Habanita* 1921
Perfumer Molinard

Ego Facto *Prends Garde à Toi* 2009
Perfumers Jean Guichard and
Aurélien Guichard

L'Artisan Parfumeur
Seville à L'Aube
Perfumer Bertrand Duchaufour

Byredo *Gypsy Water* 2008
Perfumer Jerome Epinette

Suleko *Djelem* 2013
Perfumer Cécile Zarokian

Ortigia Sicilia *Ambra Nera*
(Black Amber) 2015

Masque Milano *Tango* 2013
Perfumer Cécile Zarokian

Estée Lauder *Azurée* 1969

Sarah Horowitz Parfums
Lioness 2012
Perfumer Sarah Horowitz

CHAPTER 4
~~BEG, BORROW, OR~~ STEAL

Robert Piguet *Bandit* 1944
Perfumer Germaine Cellier

Rochas *Femme* 1943
Perfumer Edmond Roudnitska

Hermès *Calèche* 1961
Perfumer Guy Robert

Mennen (now Colgate-Palmolive)
Skin Bracer 1931

Acqua di Parma *Colonia Acqua di Parma* 1916

Comme des Garçons *Guerrilla 1*
and *Guerrilla 2* 2006
Perfumer Marie-Aude Couture-Bluche
and Nathalie Feisthaurer.

Pierre Balmain *Jolie Madame* 1953
Germaine Cellier

Revlon *That Man* 1958

Elizabeth Arden *It's You* 1938
Edmond Roudnitska

Ann Gerard *Rose Cut* 2014
Bertrand Duchaufour

Houbigant *Cologne Intense* 2015
Perfumer Luca Maffei

Amouage *Epic Woman* 2009
Perfumer Cecile Zarokian, Daniel
Maurel and Angeline Leporini

CHAPTER 4 *(continued)*
~~BEG, BORROW, OR~~ STEAL

Antonio Alessandria
Nuit Rouge 2014
Perfumer Antonio Alessandria

Jovoy Paris Lys *Epona* 2013
Perfumer Amelie Bourgeois

Comme des Garçons *Guerrilla 1*
and *Guerrilla 2* 2006
Perfumer Marie-Aude Couture-Bluche
and Nathalie Feisthaurer.

Jo Malone *Velvet Rose & Oud* 2012
Perfumer Fabrice Pellegrin

Roja Dove *Enigma* 2013
Perfumer Roja Dove

Schiaparelli *Shocking* 1937
Perfumer Jean Carles

Mont Blanc *Legend* 2011
Perfumer Olivier Pescheux

Bourjois *Evening in Paris*
(Soir de Paris) 1928
Perfumer Ernest Beaux

Evyan *Enchanting Menace* 1958

Thierry Mugler *Alien* 2005
Perfumers Dominique Ropion
and Laurent Bruyere

Azzaro *Azzaro* 1975
Perfumer Maurice Thiboud

Azzaro *Azzaro Couture* 2008
Perfumer Aurélien Guichard

Azzaro *Azzaro Pour Elle* 2015

By Kilian *Good Girls Gone Bad 2012*
Perfumer Calice Becker

Ungaro *Diva* 1983
Perfumer Jacques Polge

Juliette Has A Gun *Mad Madame* 2012
Perfumer Romano Ricci

Gucci *Envy* 1997
Perfumer Maurice Roucel

Guerlain *Jicky* 1889
Perfumer Aime Guerlain

Le Galion *Special For Gentlemen* 2014
Perfumer David Maruitte

Imaginary Authors *Memoirs of*
a Trespasser 2012
Josh Meyer

CHANEL *Sycomore* 2008
Perfumer Jacques Polge

Yves Saint Laurent *Rive Gauche* 1971
Perfumer Michel Hy

Arquiste *Boutonniere N°7* 2012
Rodrigo Flores-Roux

Yves Saint Laurent's collection
'Le Vestiaire des Parfums' series

Caban (Pea-Jacket), *Caftan, Tuxedo,*
Saharienne (bush jacket), and *Trench* 2015

Burberry *My Burberry* 2014
Perfumer Francis Kurkdjian

Ralph Lauren *Ralph Lauren Polo* 1978
Perfumer Carlos Benaim

Ramon Monegal *Cotton Musk* 2012
Perfumer Ramon Monegal

The Laundress New York

Caron *Tabac Blond* 1919
Perfumer Ernest Daltroff

Carner Barcelona *Cuirs* 2011
Perfumer Sonia Constant

Naomi Goodsir *Cuir Velours* 2012
Perfumer Julien Rasquinet

Keiko Mecheri *Lady Pointe* 2015

NICOLAÏ *Cuir Cuba Intense* 2014
Perfumer Patricia de Nicolaï

Imaginary Authors *The Cobra and the Canary* 2012 Josh Meyer

Paco Rabanne *1 Million* 2008
Perfumers Christophe Raynaud, Olivier Pescheux, and Michel Girard

Paco Rabanne *Calandre* 1969
Perfumer Michel Hy

Guerlain *Vol de Nuit* 1933
Perfumer Jacques Guerlain

Monsillage *Aviation Club* 2011
Perfumer Isabelle Michaud

Dana *Canoe* 1936
Perfumer Jean Carles

Avon *Lilac Vegetal* 1925

Revlon *Charlie!* 1973

Mary Kay *Angelfire* 1977

CHAPTER 5
THE HUNTRESS

Eau de la Reine de Hongrie
14th Century

Providence Perfume Co
Moss Gown 2012 Charna Ethier

Hermès *Amazone* 1974
Maurice Maurin

Maurer & Wirtz *Nonchalance* 1960

Hermès *Terre d'Hermès* 2006
Perfumer Jean-Claude Ellena

Jardins d'Ecrivains *Orlando* 2013
Perfumer Anaïs Biguine

The Vagabond Prince
Enchanted Forest 2012
Bertrand Duchaufour

Parfums Volnay Paris,
Brume d'Hiver 1922 /2013
Perfumer Amelie Bourgeois

Donna Karen 'Cashmere Mist' 1994

NICOLAÏ *Vie de Château Intense* 1991
Perfumer Patricia de Nicolaï

Coty *L'Origan* 1905
Perfumer François Coty

L.T. Piver *Le Trèfle Incarnat* 1898

Roger & Gallet *Vera Violetta* 1892

Guerlain *Après l'Ondée* 1906
Perfumer Jacques Guerlain

Guerlain *L'Heure Bleue* 1912
Perfumer Jacques Guerlain

Houbigant *Violette Pourpre* 1907
Perfumer Paul Parquet

D'Orsay *La Rose d'Orsay* 1908

Houbigant
Quelques Fleurs L'Original 1913
Perfumer Robert Bienaime

Rigaud *Un Air Embaumé* 1912
Marius Reboul

Floris *Edwardian Bouquet* 1901

Creed *Bois de Cedrat* 1875
Perfumer Henry Creed
Third Generation

Yardley *English Lavender* 1913

Lohse (now L'Oréal)
Uralt Lavendel 1910 Gustav Lohse

Farina
1709 Original Eau de Cologne 1709
Perfumer Johann Maria Farina

Mäurer & Wirtz
4711 Original Eau de Cologne 1792
Perfumer Wilhelm Muelhens

Acqua di Biella
Acqua di Biella N°1 1871

Ralph Lauren Safari 1990
Perfumer Dominique Ropion

Comme des Garçons Series 7 Sweet: Wood Coffee 2005

Aedes de Venustas *Cierge de Lune* 2016

CHAPTER 6 ADVANCED TECHNIQUES FOR SPECIAL PREY

Carven Ma Griffe 1946
Perfumer Jean Carles

Vivienne Westwood Libertine 2000
Perfumer Martin Gras

Frédéric Malle Portrait of a Lady 2010
Perfumer Dominique Ropion

Majda Bekkali Sculptures Olfactives Tendre Est La Nuit 2013 Delphine Thierry.

Etat Libre d'Orange Charogne (carrion) 2008
Perfumer Shyamala Maisondieu

Olfactive Studio Selfie 2015
Thomas Fontaine

Estée Lauder Youth Dew 1953
Perfumer Josephine Catapano

Elizabeth Taylor White Diamonds 1991
Perfumer Carlos Benaim

Thierry Mugler Angel 1992
Perfumer Olivier Cresp and Yves de Chirin

Prada Prada Candy 2011
Perfumer Daniela (Roche) Andrier

House Of Sillage
Passion de l'Amour 2014
Perfumer Mark Buxton

Nobile 1942 La Danza della Libellule (Dance of the Dragonflies) 2012

Calè Fragranze d'Autore
Dolce Riso 2008
Perfumer Silvio Levi

Hermès Jardin Sur le Nil 2005
Perfumer Jean-Claude Ellena

Rubini Profumi Fundamental 2015
Perfumers Cristiano Canali and Ermano Picco

Arquiste for J.Crew N°57 2015
Perfumer Carlos Huber

Arquiste for J.Crew N°31 2015
Perfumer Carlos Huber

Britney Spears Believe 2007

The Vagabond Prince Swan Princess 2014
Perfumer Bertrand Duchaufour

Marc Jacobs *Daisy* 2007
Perfumer Alberto Morillas

Lolita Lempicka
Lolita Lempicka 1997
Perfumer Annick Menardo

Room 1015 *Power Ballad* 2016
Perfumers Amélie Bourgeois and Anne-Sophie Behaghel

Yves Saint Laurent *Baby Doll* 2000
Perfumer Cécile Matton and Ralf Schwieger

Paris Hilton *Tease* 2010
Perfumer Steve Demercado

Joop! *Miss Wild* 2013
Perfumers Veronique Nyberg and Olivier Polge

Jean Patou *Huile de Chaldée* 1927
Perfumer Henri Almeras

Jean Patou *Chaldée* 1927
Perfumer Henri Almeras

Ambre-Solaire 1935 EugeneSchueller

Bain de Soleil

Coppertone 1944 Benjamin Green

Carter Wallace *Ski and Ski* 1950's
Charles Rolley

Hermes *Eau des Merveilles* 2004
Perfumers Ralf Schwieger and Nathalie Feisthauer

Bond N°9 *Fire Island* 2006
Perfumer Michel Almairac

Estée Lauder *Bronze Goddess* 2014

Guerlain Aqua Allegoria
Lys Soleia 2012
Perfumer Thierry Wasser

Carthusia *Ligea la Sirena*
Perfumer Laura Tonatto

Zarkoperfume *e'L* (2014)
Perfumer: Zarko Ahlmann Pavlov

Fragrances of Ireland *Inis* 1998
Perfumer Arthur Burnham

Givenchy *Fleur d'Interdit* 1994
Perfumer Daniel Moliere

Calvin Klein *Escape* 1993
Steve Demercado

Issey Myake *L'Eau d'Issey* 1992
Perfumer Jacques Cavallier

CB I Hate Perfume
At the Beach 1966
Perfumer Christopher Brosius

Bobby Brown *Beach* 2009

James Heeley *Sel Marin* 2008

The Different Company
Sel de Vetiver 2006
Perfumer Celine Ellena

Parfum d'Empire
Corsica Furiosa 2014
Perfumer Marc-Antoine Corticchiato

Nicolaï *Musc Monoï* 2014
Perfumer Patricia de Nicolai

Comptoir Sud Pacifique
Coco Extreme 2007

Estée Lauder *Beyond Paradise* 2003
Calice Becker

Le Galion *Sortilège* 1937/2014
Perfumer Paul Vacher/ Marie Duchene

Dana *Tabu* 1932
Perfumer Jean Carles

Nu Be *Sulphur [16S]* 2013
Perfumer Antoine Lie

Lancôme *Magie Noire* 1978
Perfumer Gerard Goupy

Calvin Klein *Obsession* 1985
Perfumer Jean Guichard

Dior *Poison* 1985
Perfumer Edouard Flechier

CHANEL *Allure 1996*
Perfumer Jacques Polge

Dior *J'Adore* 1999
Perfumer Calice Becker

Céline *Magic* 1996
Perfumers Sophia Grojsman and Alain Astori

Estée Lauder *Intuition* 2000
Perfumer Alberto Morillas

Liz Claiborne *Curve* 1996
Jean-Claude Delville

Chopard *Madness* 2001
Perfumer Christine Nagel

Unum *Opus 1144* 2015
Perfumer Filippo Sorcinelli

Rouge Bunny Rouge *Incognito* 2014
Perfumer Shyamala Maisondieu

X-Ray *Morphine* 2012

Diane Pernet *In Pursuit of Magic* 2014

Floris *Florissa* 1978

Burberry *Burberry Brit* 2003
Perfumer Nathalie Gracia-Cetto

Annick Goutal *Mandragore* 2005
Perfumers Camille Goutal in collaboration with Isabelle Doyen, the house nose.

Penhaligon's *Bluebell* 1985
Perfumer Michael Pickthall

Jo Malone *Wild Bluebell* 2011
Perfumer Christine Nagel

MiN New York *Forever Now* 2015

Philippe di Méo 'Liquides Imaginaires' *Les Eaux-Delà*

Three fragrances in this 2011 series:

Fortis Perfumer Sonia Constant

Sancti Perfumer Sonia Constant

Tumultu Perfumer Jacques Huclier

Zero Zero's *Blood Perfume* 2015

Il Profumo *Black Dianthus* 2013
Perfumer Silvana Casoli

Ulrich Lang New York
Nightscape 2009

Mark Buxton
Emotional Rescue 2013
Perfumer Mark Buxton

Puredistance *Black* 2013
Perfumer Antoine Lie

Peccato Originale (Original Sin) *Estratto di Follia*
(Extract of Madness) 2013
Perfumer Silvia Monti

Frapin *Never More* 2014
Perfumer Anne-Sophie Behaghel

Map of the Heart *Rose Heart, Red Heart, Black Heart, Gold Heart, Purple Heart* 2014-2015
Perfumer Jacques Huclier

Revlon *Intimate* 1955
Perfumer Ernest Shiftan

Prince Matchabelli
Wind Song 1953
Perfumer Ernest Shiftan

Comme des Garçons *Garage* 2004

CHAPTER 7
BAD GIRLS FANTASIES

Etat Libre d'Orange
Secretions Magnifiques
(Fabulous Secretions) 2006
Perfumer Antoine Lie

Thierry Mugler *Womanity* 2010
Perfumer Alexis Dadier

Grossmith *Hasu-no-Hana* 1888
Perfumer John Lipscomb and relaunched

2009 Perfumer Richard Melchio

Etat Libre d'Orange
Fat Electrician 2009
Perfumer Antoine Maisondieu

CHAPTER 8
MAKE WAR, NOT LOVE

Jovoy Paris *L'Art de la Guerre* 2014
Perfumer Vanina Muracciole

Caron *Narcisse Noir*
('Black Narcissus') 1911
Perfumer Ernest Daltroff

Only Brand mention:
Guerlain
Houbigant
Lubin
Grossmith
Yardley
Floris
Creed
Penhaligon's
Santa Maria Novella
Coty
L.T. Piver

Faberge BRUT 1964
Perfumer Karl Mann and Ernest Shiftan

Houbigant *Fougère Royale* 1882
Perfumer Paul Parquet

Guerlain *Mouchoir de Monsieur* 1904
Perfumer Jacques Guerlain

Coty *La Rose Jacqueminot* 1906
Perfumer François Coty

Lancôme *Poême* 1995
Perfumer Jacques Cavallier

Miller Harris *Rose en Noir* 2006
Perfumer Lyn Harris

CHANEL *Allure Homme* 1999
Jacques Polge

Malbrum *Shameless Seducer* 2015
Perfumer Delphine Thierry

Cacharel *Loulou* 1987
Perfumer Jean Guichard

Dior *Eau Sauvage* 1966
Perfumer Edmond Roudnitska

Le Galion *Paris Whip* 2014
Perfumer David Maruitte

Aether *Musk̨ethanol* 2016
Perfumers Amalie Bourgeois and
Anne-Sophie Behaghel

Knize *Knize Ten* 1924
Perfumer Vincent Roubert and
François Coty

Coty *L'Origan*
('The Golden One') 1905
Perfumer François Coty

Houbigant *Quelques Fleurs* 1912
Perfumer Robert Bienaime

Coty *Jasmin de Corse*
(jasmine of Corsica) 1906
Perfumer François Coty

Creed *Bois de Cedrat* 1875
Perfumer Henry Creed
Third Generation

Lanvin *My Sin* 1924
Perfumer "Madame Zed"

Guerlain *Après L'Ondée* 1906
Perfumer Jacques Guerlain

Aqua di Parma Colonia 1916

J.F. Schwarzlose Berlin *Treffpunkt 8 Uhr*
(Rendezvous at 8 o'clock) 2012
Perfumer Veronique Nyberg

Michael Kors *White* 2014

Lubin *Upper Ten* 2015
Perfumer Thomas Fontaine

Clinique *Happy* 1997
Perfumers Jean-Claude Delville and Rodrigo Flores-Roux

Dior *Dior Addict* 2002
Thierry Wasser

Blackbird *Pipe Bomb Intense* 2015
Perfumer Eliam Puente

Selena Gomez *Vivamore* 2013

Jennifer Lopez *Glow* 2002
Created by Louise Turner and Catherine Walsh

Christina Aguilera *Touch of Seduction* 2015

Beyoncé *Heat* 2010
Perfumers Claude Dir and Olivier Gillotin

Mariah Carey *Dreams* 2013

Katy Perry *Killer Queen* 2013
Perfumer Laurent Le Guernec

Britney Spears *Fantasy* 2005
Perfumer James Krivda

CHAPTER 9
COOL UNDER FIRE

Eau de la Reine de Hongrie
14th Century

Officina Profumo Farmaceutica Santa Maria Novella (AKA Santa Maria Novella) *Acqua della Regina* (also known as *Acqua di Colonia*) 1533

Giovanni Paolo Feminis *Aqua Admirabilis Coloniae* (Admirable Eau de Cologne) (1685-1766)

Farina 1709 *Eau de Cologne Original* 1709
Perfumer Johann Maria Farina

Mäurer & Wirtz
4711 *Eau de Cologne* 1792
Perfumer Wilhelm Muelhens

Roget & Gallet *Extra Vieille* 1806
Perfumer great-nephew of Jean-Marie Farina

Santa Maria Novella *Frangipane* 1828

Santa Maria Novella *Garofano* 1828

Santa Maria Novella *Maresciallo 1828*

Guerlain *Eau de Cologne Imperiale* 1853
Perfumer Pierre-François Pascal Guerlain

L.T. Piver
L'Eau de Cologne des Princes 1850
Perfumer Louis-Toussaint Piver

Creed *Royal Scottish Lavender* 1856
Perfumer James Henry Creed (Fifth Generation)

Creed *Jasmin Imperatrice Eugenie* 1854

House of Cleaver founded in 1770 later to become House of Yardley

Floris *Floris Limes* 1832

Floris *White Rose* 1800

Caswell-Massey *N°6* 1752
Perfumer Dr. William Hunter

Murray & Lanman *Florida Water* (sometimes known as *Kanuga Water*) 1808

Aqua di Genova
Aqua di Genova Genes 1853

Acqua di Biella
'Acqua di Biella N°1 1871

Penhaligon's *Hammam Bouquet* 1872

Two Girls a form of *Florida Water* 1908

Penhaligon's *English Fern* 1910

Aqua di Parma
Colonia Acqua di Parma 1916

Jm. Giraud Fils (Grasse-Paris)
Eau de Cologne Ambrée 1920s

Jardins de France *Oeillet* 1920s

Caron *Pour Un Homme* 1934
Perfumer Ernest Daltroff

Dunhill *Dunhill for Men* 1934

Dana *Canoe* 1936
Perfumer Jean Carles

Shulton Company *Old Spice* 1938
Perfumer Albert Hauck

Antonio Puig *Agua Lavanda* 1940

Jacques Fath *Green Water* 1947
Perfumer Vincent Roubert

Hermès *Eau d'Hermès* 1951
Perfumer Edmond Roudnitska

Dior *Eau Fraîche* 1953
Perfumer Edmond Roudnitska

Givenchy *Monsieur de Givenchy* 1959

Carven *Vetiver* 1957
Perfumer Edouard Hache

Guerlain *Vetiver* 1961
Perfumer Jean-Paul Guerlain

Givenchy *Eau de Vetyver* 1959
Perfumer Hubert Givenchy

CHANEL
CHANEL Pour Monsieur 1955
Perfumer Henri Robert

Revlon *That Man* 1958

Dior *Eau Sauvage* 1966
Perfumer Edmond Roudnitska

Lubin *Eau Neuve* (New Water) 1968
Perfumer Roger Broudoux

Santa Maria Novella *Melograno* 1965

Diptyque *L'Eau* 1968
Perfumer Desmond Knox-Leet

Bien-Être
Eau de Cologne Naturelle 1962

L'Occitane En Provence 1976
Founded by Olivier Baussan

The Body Shop
(now part of L'Oréal) 1976
Founded By Anita Roddick

Yves Saint Laurent *Pour Homme* 1971
Perfumer Raymond Chaillan

Hermès *Eau de Cologne Hermès*
(later baptized *Eau d'Orange Verte*) 1979
Françoise Caron

Diptyque *L'Ombre Dans L'Eau*
('Shadow in the water') 1983
Perfumer Serge Kalouguine

Giorgio Armani
Armani Eau Pour Homme 1984
Perfumer Roger Pellegrino

Davidoff *Cool Water* 1988
Perfumer Pierre Bourdon

Clarins *Eau Dynamisante* 1987
Perfumer Jacques Courtin-Clarins

Bath & Body Works
Founded in 1990

Elizabeth Arden *Green Tea* 1999
Perfumer Francis Kurkdjian

Jo Malone opened her first boutique 1994

Lorenzo Villoresi
Acqua di Colonia 1996

Calvin Klein *ck One* 1994
Perfumers Alberto Morillas and
Harry Fremont

Donna Karan *DKNY Women* 1999

L'Eau par Kenzo For Women 1996
Perfumer Olivier Cresp

Guerlain *Aqua Allegoria* 1999
Perfumer Jean-Paul Guerlain

Comme des Garçons
Cologne Séries 4 2002

CHANEL *Cristalle Eau Verte* 2009
Jacques Polge

Paco Rabanne
1 Million Cologne 2015
Perfumers Olivier Pescheux and
Michel Girard

Guerlain *L'Homme Ideal* EDP
in 2014 followed by *L'Homme Ideal*
Cologne in 2015
Perfumer Thierry Wasser

Thierry Mugler *Cologne* 2001
Perfumer Alberto Morillas

Cartier *L'Eau de Cartier* 2001
Perfumer Christine Nagel

Cologne Bigarde Frédéric Malle 2001
Perfumer Jean-Claude Ellena

Ralph Lauren *Blue* 2003
Perfumers David Apel and
Pierrre Negrin

Maison Francis Kurkdjian
Cologne pour la Matin 2009 and
Cologne pour le Soir 2009

Maison de Parfums Le Galion
Cologne 2015 and *Cologne Nocturne* 2016
Perfumer Rodrigo Florès-Roux

Serge Lutens *L'Eau* 2009
Perfumer Serge Lutens and
Christopher Sheldrake

Atelier Cologne *Orange Sanguine* 2010
Perfumer Ralf Schwieger

Atelier Cologne *Rose Anonyme* 2012
Perfumer Jerome Epinette

Atelier Cologne *Vétiver Fatal* 2012
Perfumer Jerome Epinette

Third Man *Eau Moderne* 2011
Perfumer Jean-Marc Chaillan

Third Man *Eau Monumentale* 2011
Perfumer Bruno Jovanovic

Third Man *Eau Profounde* 2011
Perfumer Clement Gavarry

Third Man *Eau Nomade* 2013
Perfumer Bruno Jovanovic

Frédéric Malle *Cologne Indélébile*
(Permanent Cologne) 2015
Perfumer Dominique Ropion

CHAPTER 10
THE END OF THE WORLD

Etat Libre d'Orange
La Fin Du Monde 2013
Perfumer Quentin Bisch

◈ MINI LEXICON ◈

Bad Girls Perfume Mini Lexicon

Bad Girls Perfume is deliberately not a textbook. There are, however, some terms I use throughout the book, which might not be familiar to you. Thus, this Mini-Lexicon briefly and cursorily explains or defines a few terms and expressions.

Needless to say, there are many more that I won't include here, or we'll never get out the door. Should you have questions that go beyond the scope of this lexicon, please feel free to contact me at www.badgirlsperfume.com, and I'll be happy to answer them and/or refer you to one of my favorite Bad Girls Perfume Experts.

Lexicon Table of Contents

Perfume Construction and the Perfume Pyramid

Perfume Construction
Perfume construction is often compared to musical construction with notes and chords.

Perfume Notes
Perfume notes are individual natural or synthetic raw materials, used in a fragrance composition.

Perfume Chords
Perfume chords are several notes arranged to create a single harmonic or discordant effect.

Top Notes
Top Notes are the most volatile materials in a fragrance and therefore those that evaporate in the first few minutes, giving the very first impression of the fragrance. Top notes are most often citruses, aromatic herbs (such as lavender and rosemary) and light florals.

Heart Notes
Heart Notes make up the middle part of a fragrance formula. They are what you smell after the top notes have evaporated and before the Base notes set in. Heart notes indicate the main traits of a fragrance's "personality." Heart notes can contain floral, citrus, woody, green, and musky notes.

Base Notes
Base notes are most evident in the latest stage of fragrance development after the Top and some of the Heart notes have

evaporated. Base notes are generally "heavy" such as woods, ambers, leathers, and musks.

The Perfume Pyramid

In classic perfume construction the three-tiered organization of fragrant notes is often referred to as a pyramid with base notes at the bottom, heart notes in the middle, and top notes at the summit.

Concentration Percentages of Fragrance Products

Most commercially available fragrances are composed of natural and synthetic fragrant oils in a water and alcohol base. The percentage of alcohol to water in the base can vary from 98% for perfume extracts to approximately 70% for colognes and splashes. The concentration of fragrant oils in the base can vary considerable from brand to brand. The following common percentages are included here as a useful "rule of thumb."

Pure Perfume, Perfume Extract (extrait de parfum), Perfume (parfum): 15-40% (average 25%)

Eau de Parfum: 10-20% (average 15%)

Eau de Toilette: 5-15% (average 10%)

Eau de Cologne: 3-8% (average 5%)

Cologne: up to than 4%

Splashes less than 3%

Extrait de Parfum, Parfum or Pure Perfume

Extrait de Parfum is the highest concentration of fragrant materials, containing somewhere between 15-40% , with a typical percentage being closer to 25%. It is also the most long lasting. Top notes of most volatile oils such as citrus and florals evaporate most quickly, middle notes of florals, citruses, some woods, and musks, stay on the skin longer, while the base notes may stay for twelve hours or longer.

Eau de Parfum

Eau de Parfum is generally between 10-20% of fragrant materials (average 15%), lasts longer than Eau de Toilette and has more sillage.

Eau de Toilette

Eau de Toilette is generally 5-15% (average 10%) and often includes a wider variety of fragrant materials than Eau de Cologne, such as musks, woody, and leather notes which are less volatile and therefore last longer on the skin. The word "toilette" is from the French expression for getting dressed or getting prepared to go out which is, *Faire sa toilette.*

Eau de Cologne

Eau de Cologne contains similar fragrant materials to cologne and is generally a 3-8% concentration.

Cologne

A cologne is a cocktail with a concentration of up to 4% fragrance materials in an alcohol and water base. These materials are primarily oils from the zests (rinds) of citrus fruits (lemons, limes, bergamots, oranges, and grapefruits), and can also include aromatic plants (such as rosemary and lavender), spices (such as cloves and cinnamon), as well as florals (such as roses and violets). The vast percentage of fragrant materials are highly volatile "top notes," thus evaporating and cooling very quickly with relatively little long term effect.

There can be considerable variations and overlaps in these concentrations and ingredients, and to make things more confusing, virtually all men's fragrances up until the late 1990s were referred to as "colognes" no matter what their concentration, primarily because other terms had feminine connotations.

Classification Systems

At the beginning of the 20th century perfumers saw the need for an official fragrance classification, according to dominant raw materials. The Societé Française des Parfumeurs (SFP) was the first organization to do this.

The SFP classification system

The SFP classification system divides fragrances into seven olfactory "fragrance families": Citrus, Floral, Fougère (fernlike), Oriental/Amber, Chypre, Woody, and Leather, each of which has sub-families such as "Citrus Floral," "Floral Oriental," etc.

Michael Edwards' *Fragrances of the World* "Fragrance Wheel"

Michael Edwards' *Fragrances of the World* "Fragrance Wheel" classification system was created by world renowned and respected fragrance expert and consultant, Michael Edwards. At its heart is the Fragrance Wheel, a perfume icon which defines the relationship between four "Groups" – Floral, Oriental, Woody, and Fresh – and graphically illustrates how they, in turn, evolve into fourteen individual fragrance families: Floral,

Soft Floral, Floral Oriental, Soft Oriental, Oriental, Woody Oriental, Woods, Mossy Woods, Dry Woods, Aromatic, Citrus, Water, Green (smelling of cut grass or leaves), and Fruity.

There are other classification systems, but these are the two I see used most frequently. Of course, as we all know, perfume is a living thing and as an art form is subject to individual interpretations (thank God!), which, like Bad Girls, can never be totally contained within anything so "rigid" as a classification.

I like to think of a perfume classification as a conceptual "handle" by which to grasp a fragrance and hold it in my mind in relationship with other fragrances.

In hopes of helping you do the same, I uses words from these classifications to describe fragrances in *Bad Girl Perfumes,* unless of course, the name of a fragrance does the job for me, in which case I describe it in terms of other qualities like bold, subtle, quirky, etc.

Typical Terms used in Classification Systems

Citrus

Citrus refers to the zesty smell of the rind of citrus fruits (orange, lemon, neroli, grapefruit, and bergamot) that produce a refreshing essence, and have been used in perfumery for millennia. Many perfumes and most colognes contain citrus notes.

Floral

Traditionally, floral notes are used in feminine fragrances and replicate the scent of a single flower or a bouquet of flowers.

Fougère

Fougère fragrances are primarily masculine and named after

the first *fougère* fragrance, Paul Parquet's 1882 *Fougère Royale,* built on the imaginary scent of ferns (*fougère* means fern in French). Fougère fragrances are characterized by a lavender, green, woody, and forest-y smell, and are built on the blend of lavender, oak moss and coumarin (which smells like hay, freshly mowed grass and tobacco). Fougère fragrances are often reminiscent of old school shaving lotions and creams.

Chypre

Chypre is the name of a family of fragrances, most always built around a sharp contrast of citrus notes and a woody, oak mossy accord. With a top note including bergamot, a middle note containing cistus labdanum (a resin derived from the leaves and branches cistus or "rock rose" plant), and a base note containing oak moss and patchouli. Named in honor of François Coty's 1917 fragrance *Chypre,* one of the earliest fragrances bearing this accord. Coty named his fragrance after the island of Cyprus (Chypre in French), home for many aromatic shrubs such as the rock rose, and also famous throughout antiquity for the quality of its fragrances.

Characterized as being warm and dry, mossy and animalic, chypre fragrances may also include (in addition to the basic accords), floral, fruity, other woody notes (in addition to patchouli), and leather notes.

Woody

Fragrances that smell warm and opulent like sandalwood and patchouli, or dry like cedar and vetiver.

Oriental/Amber

Hot and sultry, oriental/amber fragrances are dominant and

overpowering, typically smelling of amber, resins, vanilla, incense, spices, amber, and oud. They are called "orientals" because they evoke smells that westerners associate with India, the Middle East and the Far East.

Leather

The smallest group of fragrances, leathers, are dry, sometimes very dry notes, sometimes luxurious and sometimes tough, and meant to evoke the smell of leather or elements associated with leather tanning and preparation, such as smoke, burnt wood, honey, wood, and wood tars or tobacco.

Gourmand

Gourmand fragrances are not considered a family or group in their own right in either the SFP Classification, or in Michael Edwards' Fragrance Wheel. For example, in the SFP classification, *Angel* is classified as a "Floral Woody Amber," while in Michael Edwards' classification, *Angel* is classified as a "Woody Oriental." Gourmand fragrances typically contain significant edible or food smelling notes such as vanilla, candy, tonka beans, honey, chocolate, berries, cinnamon, cupcakes, whiskey, sugared almond and marzipan, even cotton candy or coffee. The French term "Gourmand" is often used to refer to a person with a sweet tooth.

Green

Smelling of cut grass or leaves

Aromatic

The term aromatic can be confusing because in French it refers to any fragrant substance, while in English it often refers specifically to the sharp pungent fragrance of herbs such as lavender, sage, rosemary, etc.

A Few Significant Raw Materials Definitions and Usages

Plant Products

Amber

Amber is a general term referring to any number of fragrant blends made of resins such as styrax, benzoin, and cistus labdanum. (See specific definitions of these resins.) Ambers are associated with fragrances of the Middle East and therefore one of the characteristic ingredients of "Oriental" fragrances.

Benzoin

Benzoin is an oil with a pleasantly antiseptic smell reminiscent of vanilla, and is extracted from a Styrax Benzoin tree. In addition to its medicinal value as an antiseptic, benzoin is a common ingredient in incense and perfumes and is associated with "Oriental" fragrances.

Bergamot

A citrus fruit typical of Mediterranean regions that is slightly larger than a lemon and smaller than an orange. The distinctive smell of Earl Gray tea comes from bergamot.

Galbanum

Galbanum is a plant resin with a bitter green smell, associated with oriental fragrances.

Labdanum

Labdanum or Cistus Labdanum is a resin or amber obtained from the leaves and branches of the ciste plant, a flowering shrub that grows in Mediterranean regions. Cistus Labdanum has the sweet, woody, somewhat leathery smell often associates with churches and/or polished woods. Cistus Labdanum is part of the basic formula for chypre fragrances, and also common in oriental and fougère fragrances.

Oak moss

Oak moss is a tree material with a distinctive bitter smell and is part of the distinctive scent of chypre fragrances.

Oud

Oud, also known as Agarwood is an aromatic resinous substance that forms in evergreen Aquilaria and Gyrinops trees native to southeast Asia when they have been infected with a certain type of mold. Oud is valued for its distinctive scent characterized as soft fruity, floral, woody, and balsamic with shades of vanilla, musk, and, ambergris. Oud has been used in perfumery since antiquity, and has enjoyed renewed popularity especially in the 21st century in oriental-amber fragrances.

Patchouli

Patchouli is a green busy herb that grows mainly in India. The leaves are used in perfumery for their pungent sweet, dark, and earthy aroma. Because of its use as an insecticide in the transportation of exotic cloths from India to France in the 19th century, it became associated with Belle Epoque prostitutes. In the 20th century during the 60s and 70s, it became associated with hippies and flower children of the Sexual Revolution because of its ties with India and the Hare Krishna movement. Today, it has found its place as a green and erotic note in classy, high-end fragrances.

Resin

A resin is a thick plant extract of similar consistency to molasses. Typical resins used in perfumery are cistus labdanum, benzoin, and galbanum.

Vetiver

Vetiver is dry "beach grass" whose fragrant root is used in perfumery. Its odor is dry-edged, green, and earthy, and recalls the mellow brown of a cigar or beautifully tanned leather. There's also a brightness to it, and a saltiness that makes me think of straw hats, beach mats, and sunshine. Traditionally used primarily in men's fragrances, it is increasingly finding its way into Bad Girls territory. Thank goodness. It's one of my favorite raw materials.

Animal Products

Animal products were used in traditional perfumery for their erotic animalistic smells and also as fixatives for the other fragrant materials. Because of heightened concerns for animal rights among the general public they are seldom used in modern perfumery, and their odors have been replaced with synthetic molecules.

Ambergris

Ambergris is regurgitation (vomit) from sperm whales, which having floated and ripened for months or years on the sea, is washed up on shore. Ambergris is highly prized for it erotic odor and strong fixative qualities when used in perfumery.

Musk

Musk is obtained by surgical removal from the "musk pod" (near sexual organs) of the Himalayan musk deer.

Civet

Civet is dander scraped from the hairs of civet cats.

Synthetics

Contemporary Bad Girls are heirs to the chemical discoveries that were taking place in Europe during the second half of the 19th century (right around the time Scarlet O'Hara was carrying out her numerous Bad Girl Schemes), and were to have game changing impact on the world wide perfume industry. The development of synthetic fragrance molecules, such as coumarin in 1868 (which smells like newly mown hay), vanillin in 1874, which smells like vanilla, the first synthetic musk in 1888, and ionone in 1893, the odorous principle of violets. Perfumers realized that synthetic molecules could be useful in fragrance compositions because they offered specific scents otherwise unavailable or difficult to obtain in nature. Additionally, some synthetics (such as aldehydes) highlight the natural molecules in a formula for a totally new olfactory delivery.

The first fragrance to include synthetic molecules in its composition was Houbigant's *Fougère Royale* in 1882. Others were soon to follow, notably Guerlain's *Jicky* in 1889.

The significance of synthetics for fragrance compositions is that they allowed perfumers to create with fragrant notes beyond the natural realm. This can be compared to the availability of portable paint tubes for artists of approximately the same period, which allowed them to paint outside instead of in studios. Both phenomena opened the way to enormous potential of "abstract" creations.

Indeed, it can be argued that it is thanks to the infinite possibilities synthetics bring to the perfumer's palette that fragrance composition evolved from a "craft" to an "art" at the time, and the growth and importance of the perfume industry literally exploded at the beginning of the 20th century. Today, the vast majority of fragrances include synthetics.

Aldehydes

Aldehydes are organic chemical compounds. The best known of the aldehydes are C10, C11, and C12, which were made famous in CHANEL N°5. Although known for the variety and intensity of their smells, aldehydes are especially appreciated in perfume compositions because of their capacity to enhance and boost ("stir up") the fragrance and diffusion of other raw materials in a formula, for a "shimmering" and "effervescent" delivery.

Calone

Calone is a synthetic raw material evoking the smell of fresh melon as well as the ethereal, ozon-y sensation of breaking waves, sea-breezes, and marine life. Calone is often used in marine or "aquatic" fragrances.

Coumarin

A fragrant molecule used in perfumery to add a sweet note suggestive of freshly mown hay or cut grass. In nature it is found in Tonka Beans which grow on cumaru trees, and it can also be produced synthetically. First developed in the late 19th Century, synthetic coumarin was one of the first synthetic molecules to be used in perfumery, and was therefore part of the first exciting steps in modern perfumery, which dared to mix synthetic raw materials with naturals.

Musks Old and New

Classic old musk fragrance materials are derived from animal products that are now banned, or so costly that they are rarely used in modern perfumery. These natural musks have animalic smells (like animals), and are characterized as "erotic," or "dirty."

Synthetic musks are also known as white musks. Although they imitate the odor of deer musk and add sensual and erotic elements to perfumes, they do not have the fecal smell of natural musks, and instead smell clean and airy – like freshly laundered and line-dried bed linens or like clean skin. Most, if not all musks used in perfumery today are synthetic.

A Few Other Perfume Terms

Animalic

This term is often used loosely to describe a fragrance which suggests animal or bodily smells. They may be sensual, perhaps musky, sweaty, or dirty (in the sense of dirty underwear). They are often found in the base notes or "dry-down" of a fragrance. In traditional perfume, animalic smells were created by the addition of musk, castoreum, civet, or ambergris.

The Fragrance Foundation

The Fragrance Foundation, established in 1949, is a non-profit organization whose membership includes more than 82 of the world's most important corporations in the fragrance industry. Each year the Fragrance Foundation presents awards, fondly known as "FiFi" Awards, to celebrate achievements in perfumery. Fragrance Foundation "Fifi" Awards are the fragrance industry equivalent of Academy Award "Oscars" for the film industry.

Sillage

This French term literally means the wake that a passing boat leaves in water. In perfumery it refers to the fragrance "trail" that lingers in the air or in memory after the wearer has gone, and is often used in English because there is not an equivalent term that specifically describes this phenomenon.

Denatured Alcohol

Thanks to modern, supposedly protective (read Bad Girl "kill joy") global norms and regulations, the alcohol components in all commercially sold cologne and perfume products have been "denatured," i.e., made to taste and digest horribly.

Non-Perfumery Terms and References

Au contraire

Au contraire is a French term meaning, "on the contrary."

BoBo

BoBo is a French term that stands for "Bourgeois Bohemian," and means a person who combines a bourgeois, affluent lifestyle with a bohemian way of life.

Chercher quelqu'un

Chercher quelqu'un is a French expression that literally means, "to go out looking for somebody," but the expression is similar to "egging somebody on," or "trying to get a rise out of them by pushing their buttons."

Doyenne

A doyenne is a powerful woman, particularly in the art world.

In extremis

In extremis is a Latin expression meaning, "in extreme circumstances."

Je ne sais quoi

Je ne sais quoi is a French term meaning, "that indefinable something."

Ménage à trois

Ménage à trois is a French expression referring to three people (often a woman with two men) living together.

Mine de rien

Mine de rien is a French expression that means, "innocent looking."

Pour la petite histoire

Pour la petite histoire is a French expression that means something like, "to fill you in on the back-story" and is similar to the current expression, FYI.

Quand même

Quand même is a French expression meaning, "Indeed!" or "What the hell!"

Terroire

Terroire is a French word meaning, "native land or territory."

End

◈ ACKNOWLEDGEMENTS ◈

As I reach the end of this book project that has lasted almost three years I am grateful to my husband, Pierre, who helped and encouraged me from the very beginning, as always, even when he didn't have a clue what I was doing.

My three daughters, Elisabeth, Catherine, and Florence, were right there for the entire experience as well, and depending upon the needs of the moment have served as faithful and capable editors, producers, cheerleaders, bar tenders, midwives, and shrinks.

Adelaide Farah has been my mentor and friend since 1999 when she hired me as Paris Correspondent for *Beauty Fashion* magazine (perfume and cosmetics), so after listening to my ideas, advising, and encouraging me for years, it seemed natural that she would accept the job of editing *Bad Girls Perfume.* Even so, neither she nor I could have known what a sometimes hair raising, sometimes exhausting, always thrilling adventure this would be. The fruit of our teamwork goes far beyond the accomplishment of publishing a book.

Meanwhile, my friends Karen Marin, Silvio Lévi, and Uli Lang have been more than the perfect and faithful friends for every aspect of this project.

Offering technical support and encouragement, for this book and over the years, perfumers Shyamala Maisondieu, Patricia de Nicolaï, Jean Kerléo, Thomas Fontaine, Amalie Bourgeois, and Anne-Sophie Behaghel have been heroes.

For historical support, Annick Le Guérer, perfume historian *par excellence,* has offered guidance and information, while Isabelle Ferrand, CEO and owner of Cinquième Sens generously shared research on trends in perfumes and colognes.

The cover design was a joint effort starting with Jocelyn Haybittel Gibson who totally got the idea of *Bad Girls Perfume* and created the Bad Girl Devil image and perfume bottle first crack out of the box. Helder Suffenplan gave me advice about aesthetics, Pamela Paddock helped me play with first drafts in Photoshop, and Catherine Villeminot brought the whole front cover together for a dynamic design and message. Meanwhile, graphic artist, Catherine Seris, designed the back cover and integrated both front and back covers for a witty and coherent whole.

Catherine Seris was also creative, calm, and assured as she guided me through layout and into the printing process.

Charter member Bad Boys of my first official Bad Girls Perfume Party in Paris will always have a special place in my heart: Etienne de Swardt, Thomas Lindet, Jean-Claude Magret, Antoine Lie, Wouter Wiels, Abraham de Amézaga, Quentin Bisch, and Pierre Villeminot.

Astrologer Muriel Siron, played an essential role in first pointing out that my Bad Girl stars, planets, and cards were perfectly aligned for this project, and then guiding me through the process of making it happen.

Friends and family, inside and outside the fragrance industry, have inspired and amused me by setting high standards for Bad Girl and Bad Boy behavior as they go about their everyday Action Hero lives. To name just a few, and in random order: Nicolas Chabot, Cassandra Moonen-Ferrera, Judy Davis, Kate Bourdet, DG Martin, Gilles Thévenin, Landon Nordeman, Sophie Cauchi, Patrick Saint Yves, François Hénin, Etienne de Swardt, Karl Brandl, Robert Gerstner, Manon Carrere, Nicolas Cloutier, David Frossard, Prudence Kilgour, Neela Vermeire, Antonio de Figueiredo, Michael Edwards, Joe Garces, Céline Tréhet, Arnaud Guggenbuhl, François Duquesne, Céleste Duquesne, Jan Moran, Susan Lewis, Pascal Guasp, Saskia Wilson-Brown, Kathryn Malley, Ala Zander, Rossella Caputo, Raphaella Barkley, The SOTs (Farley, Twig, Pooh, Paula, and Bacot), Berna Huebner, Anna Hayes, Millie Cox, DeDe Caughman, Josh O'Donovan, Eleanor Owen, Sallie Chaballier, Deborah Lillian, Karen Hartman, Sallie Lee, Meg Lee, Carol Britt Porter, Sallie Broach, Nancy Brune, Jane Mobille, Claude de Calbiac, the entire Grassroots team, especially Kelly Reuba and Michele Rumfola, Ann Henaff, Whitney de Courcel, Margarita Battle, Byron Battle, Mayla Castillo, Marie Colton, Liz Colton, Marie Colton Woodard, and Walter Colton.

Writings by members of the perfume community in the form of books, blogs, websites, and newsletters have been indispensible for this book. In a world of internet connections it is a pleasure to know that in addition to their works I know most of these people personally through interactions in Paris or at international perfume trade shows such as, Esxence in Milan, Pitti in Florence, Elements and NYNOW in New York, and most recently, Tranoï in Paris.

Books

Annick Le Guérer *Le Parfum*

Bettina Aykroyd *Les Énigmes du Parfum*

Chandler Burr *The Perfect Scent* and other books and articles

Dariush Alavi *Perfume Le Snob*

Denyse Beaulieu *The Perfume Lover*

Elisabeth de Feydeau *Les Parfums*

Jean-Claude Ellena *Journal d'un Parfumeur* and other books

Luca Turin *Perfumes: The A-Z Guide* and other books

Lindy Woodhead *War Paint*

Michael Edwards *Perfume Legends*

Osmothèque and Annick Le Guérer *Once Upon A Time…Perfume*

Osmothèque, Sabine Chabbert, and Laurence Férat *Rare Perfumes*

Société Française des Parfumeurs *Official Fragrance Catalogue and Terminology*

Tilar J. Mazzeo *The Secret of CHANEL NO.5*

Websites, Blogs and Newsletters

Bettina Aykroyd *Faire Le Tour Du Monde En Parfums*

Clayton Ilolahia *What Men Should Smell Like*

CosmétiqueMag

Dariush Alavi *Persolaise*

Denyse Beaulieu *Grain de Musc*

Elena Knezhevich and Zoran Knezevic *Fragrantica*

Elisabeth de Feydeau's *News*

Ermano Picco *La Gardenia nell'Occhiello*

Helder Suffenplan *Scentury*

Jo Fairley and Lorna McKay *The Perfume Society*

Mark Behnke *Colognoisseur*

Méchant Loup / Thierry Blondeau *Olfactorum*

Megan Paki *Megan In Sainte Maxime*

Michelyn Camen *Ça Fleure Bon*

Oonagh Phillips *BW Confidential*

Nathalie Pichard *Topnotes*

Michael Edwards *Fragrances of the World (Year Books)*

Ozmoz

Patricia de Nicolaï *Nicolaï*

Patty White *Perfume Posse*

Robin Krug *Now Smell This*

Sophie Normand *My Blue Hour*

Victoria Frolova *Bois de Jasmin*

WWD

End

Achevé d'imprimer en mars 2016 par
Créaprojet, 7 rue François Mortureux, 21200 Beaune
Dépôt légal : mars 2016
Numéro d'impression : 119825
Imprimé en France